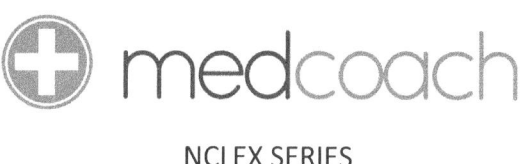

NCLEX SERIES

NCLEX-RN Practice Exam Part 1:
150 MCQs With Detailed Answers and Explanations

MedCoach 2023

Table of Contents

Question 1 17
    Topic: Implementing Advance Directives 18

Question 2 20
    Topic: Delegation and Supervision in Client Care 21

Question 3 23
    Topic: Cost-Effective Care Strategies 24

Question 4 25
    Topic: Client Plan of Care Evaluation and Updating 26

Question 5 28
    Topic: Education on Client Rights and Responsibilities 29

Question 6 31
    Topic: Advocacy for Client Rights and Needs 32

Question 7 34
    Topic: Collaboration with a Multi-Disciplinary Team 35

Question 8 37
    Topic: Effective Time Management in Nursing 38

Question 9 39
    Topic: Conflict Management in Healthcare 40

Question 10 42
    Topic: Maintaining Client Confidentiality and Privacy 43

Question 11 45
    Topic: Handoff of Care Reporting 46

Question 12 48
    Topic: Approved Terminology in Documenting Care 49

Question 13 51
    Topic: Safe Admission, Transfer, and Discharge Procedures 52

Question 14 54
    Topic: Prioritizing Care Based on Acuity 55

Question 15 57
    Topic: Ethical Dilemmas in Nursing 58

Question 16 60
    Topic: Nurses' Code of Ethics 61

Question 17 62
    Topic: Client Education and Consent for Care 63

Question 18 65
    Topic: Implementation of Healthcare Provider Orders 66

Question 19 68
    Topic: Utilizing Resources for Quality Client Care 69

Question 20 71
    Topic: Recognizing and Reporting Limitations of Self and Others . 72

Question 21 74
    Topic: Reporting Client Conditions as Required by Law 75

Question 22 77
    Topic: Legal Scope of Nursing Practice 78

Question 23 80
    Topic: Participation in Performance Improvement Projects 81

Question 24 82
    Topic: Assessing the Need for Referrals 83

Question 25 84
    Topic: Allergy Assessment and Intervention 85

Question 26 86
    Topic: Client Care Environment Assessment 87

Question 27 88
    Topic: Promoting Staff Safety 89

Question 28 91
    Topic: Client Injury Prevention 92

Question 29 93
    Topic: Client Identification Procedures 94

Question 30 95
    Topic: Verification of Treatment Order Appropriateness 96

Question 31 97
    Topic: Emergency Planning and Response 98

Question 32 100
    Topic: Using Ergonomic Principles in Care 101

Question 33 103
    Topic: Handling Biohazardous and Hazardous Materials 104

Question 34 106
    Topic: Client Safety Education 107

Question 35 109
    Topic: Documenting Practice Errors and Near Misses 110

Question 36 111
    Topic: Reporting Unsafe Practice of Healthcare Personnel 112

Question 37 114
    Topic: Safe Use of Equipment 115

Question 38 116
    Topic: Implementing Security Plans and Procedures 117

Question 39 119
    Topic: Infection Prevention Principles 120

Question 40 122
    Topic: Educating on Infection Prevention Measures 123

Question 41 124
    Topic: Use of Restraints 125

Question 42 126
    Topic: Care for Newborns, Infants, and Toddlers 127

Question 43 128
    Topic: Care for Preschool and School Age Clients 129

Question 44 130
    Topic: Care for Adult Clients (18-64 years) 131

Question 45 132
    Topic: Care for Geriatric Clients (65+ years) 133

Question 46 135
    Topic: Prenatal Care and Education 136

Question 47 138
    Topic: Antepartum and Labor Client Care 139

Question 48 .... **141**
    Topic: Post-Partum Care and Education 142

Question 49 .... **144**
    Topic: Health Risk Assessments Based on Family, Community ... 145

Question 50 .... **147**
    Topic: Learning Readiness, Preferences, and Barriers Assessment 148

Question 51 .... **149**
    Topic: Community Health Education 150

Question 52 .... **152**
    Topic: Preventative Care and Health Maintenance 153

Question 53 .... **155**
    Topic: Communication Barrier Minimization 156

Question 54 .... **158**
    Topic: Targeted Screening Assessments 159

Question 55 .... **160**
    Topic: High Risk Health Behavior Prevention and Treatment 161

Question 56 .... **162**
    Topic: Managing Care in Home Environment 163

Question 57 .... **164**
    Topic: Comprehensive Health Assessments 165

Question 58 .... **167**
    Topic: Assessing for Abuse or Neglect 168

Question 59 .... **170**

Topic: Behavioral Management Techniques in Care 171

Question 60 173

Topic: Substance Abuse Assessment and Intervention 174

Question 61 176

Topic: Coping with Life Changes 177

Question 62 179

Topic: Violence Potential Assessment and Safety Precautions ... 180

Question 63 182

Topic: Incorporating Cultural Practices in Care 183

Question 64 185

Topic: End-of-Life Care and Education 186

Question 65 188

Topic: Assessing Client Support System 189

Question 66 191

Topic: Providing Care for Grieving Clients 192

Question 67 194

Topic: Acute and Chronic Psychosocial Health Issues 195

Question 68 197

Topic: Psychosocial Factors Influencing Care 198

Question 69 200

Topic: Caring for Clients with Sensory or Cognitive Alterations .. 201

Question 70 203

Topic: Recognizing Non-Verbal Cues to Stressors 204

Question 71 206

Topic: Using Therapeutic Communication Techniques 207

Question 72 209

Topic: Promoting a Therapeutic Environment 210

Question 73 212

Topic: Assisting Clients with Physical or Sensory Impairments ... 213

Question 74 215

Topic: Management of Bowel and Bladder Alteration 216

Question 75 218

Topic: Performing Irrigations 219

Question 76 221

Topic: Skin Integrity Maintenance 222

Question 77 224

Topic: Orthopedic Devices Application and Maintenance 225

Question 78 227

Topic: Measures to Promote Circulation 228

Question 79 230

Topic: Pain Assessment and Intervention 231

Question 80 233

Topic: Evidence-based Complementary Therapies for Pain Management 234

Question 81 236

Topic: Positioning for Comfort and Safety 237

Question 82 239

Topic: Assisting with Invasive Procedures 240

Question 83 242
    Topic: Implementing and Monitoring Phototherapy 243

Question 84 245
    Topic: Maintaining Optimal Temperature of Client 246

Question 85 248
    Topic: Monitoring and Caring for Clients on a Ventilator 249

Question 86 251
    Topic: Drainage Device Monitoring and Maintenance 252

Question 87 254
    Topic: Peritoneal Dialysis Performance and Management 255

Question 88 257
    Topic: Performing Suctioning 258

Question 89 260
    Topic: Wound Care and Dressing Change 261

Question 90 263
    Topic: Providing Ostomy Care and Education 264

Question 91 266
    Topic: Providing Pulmonary Hygiene 267

Question 92 269
    Topic: Postoperative Care Provision 270

Question 93 272
    Topic: Fluid and Electrolyte Imbalance Management 273

Question 94 276
    Topic: Arterial Line Monitoring and Maintenance 277

Question 95 279
  Topic: Pacing Device Care Management 280

Question 96 282
  Topic: Telemetry Client Care Management 283

Question 97 285
  Topic: Hemodialysis or Continuous Renal Replacement Therapy Care Management 286

Question 98 288
  Topic: Care of Clients with Hemodynamic, Tissue Perfusion, and Hemostasis Alterations 289

Question 99 291
  Topic: Education Regarding Acute or Chronic Conditions 292

Question 100 294
  Topic: Management of Clients with Impaired Ventilation/Oxygenation 295

Question 101 297
  Topic: Evaluating Effectiveness of Treatment Plan for Acute or Chronic Diagnosis 298

Question 102 300
  Topic: Performing Emergency Care Procedures 301

Question 103 303
  Topic: Pathophysiology Related to Acute or Chronic Conditions 304

Question 104 306
  Topic: Recognizing Signs and Symptoms of Client Complications 307

Question 105 309
  Topic: Intervening as Needed for Client Complications 310

Question 106 312
   Topic: Cardiovascular System Disorders 313

Question 107 315
   Topic: Respiratory System Disorders 316

Question 108 318
   Topic: Musculoskeletal System Disorders 319

Question 109 321
   Topic: Integumentary System Disorders 322

Question 110 324
   Topic: Gastrointestinal System Disorders 325

Question 111 327
   Topic: Endocrine System Disorders 328

Question 112 330
   Topic: Genitourinary System Disorders 331

Question 113 333
   Topic: Immune System Disorders 334

Question 114 336
   Topic: Nervous System Disorders 337

Question 115 339
   Topic: Hematological Disorders 340

Question 116 342
   Topic: Eye Disorders 343

Question 117 345
   Topic: Ear Disorders 346

Question 118 .... **348**
    Topic: Nose, Mouth, and Throat Disorders 349

Question 119 .... **351**
    Topic: Reproductive System Disorders 352

Question 120 .... **354**
    Topic: Pregnancy and Childbirth Related Disorders 355

Question 121 .... **357**
    Topic: Newborn and Infant Disorders 358

Question 122 .... **360**
    Topic: Pediatric Disorders 361

Question 123 .... **363**
    Topic: Elderly Client Disorders 364

Question 124 .... **366**
    Topic: Pharmacological Pain Management 367

Question 125 .... **369**
    Topic: Non-Pharmacological Pain Management 370

Question 126 .... **372**
    Topic: Common Drug Interactions 373

Question 127 .... **375**
    Topic: Client Education on Drug Side Effects and Adherence 376

Question 128 .... **378**
    Topic: Assessing Client Understanding of Drug Therapy 379

Question 129 .... **381**
    Topic: Medication Error Prevention 382

Question 130 .... **384**
Topic: Medication Reconciliation 385

Question 131 .... **387**
Topic: Administration of Parenteral Medications 388

Question 132 .... **390**
Topic: Administration of Enteral Medications 391

Question 133 .... **393**
Topic: Administration of Topical Medications 394

Question 134 .... **396**
Topic: Administration of Inhalation Medications 397

Question 135 .... **399**
Topic: Administration of Transdermal Medications 400

Question 136 .... **402**
Topic: Over the Counter Drug Education and Safety 403

Question 137 .... **405**
Topic: Monitoring Therapeutic Drug Levels 406

Question 138 .... **408**
Topic: Nutritional Therapy Implementation 409

Question 139 .... **411**
Topic: Food and Drug Interactions 412

Question 140 .... **413**
Topic: Parenteral Nutrition Administration 414

Question 141 .... **416**
Topic: Enteral Feeding Administration 417

Question 142 .... **419**
    Topic: Nutritional Assessment and Client Education 420

Question 143 .... **422**
    Topic: Dietary Supplements and Herbal Remedies 423

Question 144 .... **425**
    Topic: Assisting with Activities of Daily Living 426

Question 145 .... **428**
    Topic: Physical Mobility Promotion 429

Question 146 .... **431**
    Topic: Use of Assistive Devices 432

Question 147 .... **434**
    Topic: Home Safety Education 435

Question 148 .... **437**
    Topic: Exercise and Activity Education 438

Question 149 .... **440**
    Topic: Rehabilitation and Restorative Care 441

Question 150 .... **442**
    Topic: Pre-Operative and Post-Operative Care 443

Looking for more practice? **445**

Question 1

The nurse is caring for a client who has an advance directive in place. The client's daughter is present and requests the nurse to perform a procedure that contradicts the directive.

What should the nurse do?
1. Follow the daughter's request.
2. Seek advice from the nursing manager.
3. Follow the instructions in the advance directive.
4. Seek legal advice.

Answer Key
Option 3

Topic: Implementing Advance Directives

In the context of the NCLEX exam, understanding and implementing advance directives is crucial. Advance directives are legal documents that allow patients to convey their decisions about end-of-life care ahead of time. They provide a way for patients to communicate their wishes to family, friends, and health care professionals, and to avoid confusion later on. These directives usually encompass a living will and a durable power of attorney for health care.

The NCLEX exam tests your ability to prioritize and make decisions that respect patient autonomy, are ethically sound, and abide by legal guidelines. In the given question, despite the daughter's request, the nurse is ethically and legally bound to adhere to the client's wishes as stated in the advance directive. The principle of patient autonomy supersedes family desires or medical team recommendations. This is particularly important in end-of-life situations or when patients cannot express their wishes themselves.

When preparing for the NCLEX, familiarize yourself with the ethical principles of nursing practice, such as autonomy, beneficence, nonmaleficence, and justice. Practice various scenarios involving ethical dilemmas and understand the laws around healthcare decision-making, such as the Patient Self-

Determination Act, which encourages individuals to think about and document their future healthcare wishes.

Question 2

The charge nurse on a medical-surgical floor is making assignments at the beginning of the shift. Which of the following tasks should the charge nurse delegate to a licensed practical nurse (LPN)?

1. Teaching a newly diagnosed diabetic patient how to administer insulin.
2. Initiating a blood transfusion for a patient with a low hemoglobin level.
3. Administering a scheduled dose of oral medication for a patient with hypertension.
4. Conducting a cognitive assessment for a patient with a suspected stroke.

Answer Key

The correct answer is: 3. Administering a scheduled dose of oral medication for a patient with hypertension.

Topic: Delegation and Supervision in Client Care

When studying for the NCLEX, it's essential to understand the scope of practice for different healthcare providers. In this case, the question focuses on what tasks can be safely and appropriately delegated to a Licensed Practical Nurse (LPN).

The charge nurse, who is a Registered Nurse (RN), is responsible for making appropriate patient assignments that take into account the scope of practice for each staff member. In many settings, an LPN's scope of practice includes administering oral medications, making this the correct answer.

Option 1 is incorrect because patient teaching, especially for critical skills such as insulin administration, is typically the responsibility of the RN. Option 2 is also not suitable for delegation to an LPN because initiating a blood transfusion requires advanced assessment and intervention skills. Lastly, conducting cognitive assessments (option 4) generally falls within the RN's scope of practice as it involves complex data interpretation and decision-making.

Preparing for this type of question on the NCLEX requires a solid understanding of the scope of practice for different roles in the healthcare team. It would be beneficial to review the nurse practice acts or regulations in your region or country, which usually outline what each role can do. Moreover, engaging in exercises or case studies that require delegation decisions can be incredibly useful in honing these skills for the NCLEX exam.

Question 3

A nurse manager is conducting a team meeting to discuss cost-effective care strategies. Which of the following suggestions made by a team member should the nurse manager consider implementing?

1. Using the newest, most expensive medical equipment for all procedures.
2. Ordering duplicate laboratory tests to confirm diagnoses.
3. Implementing a protocol for regular maintenance of equipment.
4. Encouraging patients to stay longer in the hospital for more thorough care.

Answer Key

The correct answer is: 3. Implementing a protocol for regular maintenance of equipment.

Topic: Cost-Effective Care Strategies

In the context of the NCLEX exam, understanding cost-effective care strategies is crucial as it focuses on efficient and sustainable use of healthcare resources without compromising quality patient care.

In the given question, option 3 is the correct answer because regular maintenance of equipment can prevent breakdowns, extend the equipment's lifespan, and prevent costly emergency repairs or replacements. It's a cost-effective strategy that promotes patient safety and supports uninterrupted healthcare delivery.

Option 1 is not cost-effective as newer, more expensive equipment is not always necessary and can inflate costs without improving patient outcomes. Option 2 suggests ordering duplicate tests, which is usually unnecessary and may lead to wasteful spending. Lastly, option 4 is also not cost-effective; extended hospital stays can increase healthcare costs without necessarily improving patient outcomes. Instead, focusing on timely, quality care and discharge planning is more cost-effective.

Question 4

A nurse is evaluating the plan of care for a client who was admitted with a fractured hip and has undergone surgery. Which of the following actions should the nurse take to accurately evaluate and update the client's plan of care?

1. Wait until the client is ready for discharge to reassess the effectiveness of the plan of care.
2. Continue with the same interventions, even if the client's condition changes.
3. Evaluate the client's progress toward goals and update the plan of care as necessary.
4. Delegate the task of updating the care plan to a nursing assistant.

Answer Key

The correct answer is: 3. Evaluate the client's progress toward goals and update the plan of care as necessary.

Topic: Client Plan of Care Evaluation and Updating

On the NCLEX exam, understanding how to effectively evaluate and update a client's plan of care is fundamental. This knowledge reflects the ability to provide dynamic, patient-centered care based on ongoing assessments and evolving patient needs.

In the provided question, option 3 is the correct answer because it emphasizes the importance of continually evaluating a client's progress toward the established goals and adjusting the plan of care as needed. This ensures the care provided remains relevant and effective for the client's current condition.

Option 1 is incorrect as waiting until discharge to reassess the effectiveness of the plan of care would be too late to make necessary adjustments. Regularly evaluating and updating the care plan ensures timely, effective interventions.

Option 2 is not appropriate as sticking to the same interventions regardless of the client's condition doesn't consider the dynamic nature of patient needs and could lead to ineffective care.

Option 4 is not correct because although delegation is an important nursing skill, the task of evaluating and updating a care plan requires the critical thinking and clinical judgment skills of a registered nurse.

To prepare for NCLEX, it's crucial to understand the importance of continuous evaluation and updating of the care plan. Be familiar with the process of assessment, setting measurable goals, implementing interventions, and evaluating outcomes. This cyclical process ensures the delivery of individualized and effective nursing care.

Question 5

The nurse is preparing to provide education on client rights and responsibilities to a client who has been recently diagnosed with type 2 diabetes. Which of the following statements should the nurse include in the teaching?

1. "You have the right to refuse any treatment, even if it might negatively affect your health."
2. "Your responsibility is to follow all the instructions provided by the healthcare team without questioning."
3. "As a client, you are not allowed to request a different healthcare provider if you are unsatisfied with your current one."
4. "You don't have the right to know the risks and benefits of treatments before you decide to accept them."

Answer Key

The correct answer is: 1. "You have the right to refuse any treatment, even if it might negatively affect your health."

Topic: Education on Client Rights and Responsibilities

In the NCLEX examination, there's an emphasis on understanding client rights and responsibilities, which includes their right to informed consent and the right to refuse care or treatment.

In the question provided, option 1 is the correct answer because it accurately represents a fundamental client right, which is the right to refuse any treatment, even if it may negatively affect their health. This right is protected by law and ensures that the client has autonomy and control over their healthcare decisions.

Option 2 is incorrect. While clients have the responsibility to follow healthcare instructions to maintain their health, they also have the right to question or seek clarification about any aspect of their care. It encourages active participation in care and decision making.

Option 3 is not accurate. Clients have the right to request a different healthcare provider if they're unsatisfied with their current one, as part of their right to have a say in their healthcare.

Option 4 is also incorrect. Clients have the right to be informed about the risks and benefits of treatments before deciding to accept them, known as informed consent.

To prepare for the NCLEX, it's important to understand the rights and responsibilities of clients. This includes the right to refuse care, the right to privacy and confidentiality, the right to be informed, the right to choose their healthcare provider, and the right to have their pain effectively managed. Equally important is the understanding of client responsibilities, which include providing accurate information to the healthcare team, following the treatment plan, and communicating changes in health status.

Question 6

A nurse is caring for a client who is hard of hearing and English is not their first language. The client's family insists on translating and refuses the use of a professional interpreter. What is the most appropriate action for the nurse to take?

1. Allow the family to translate to make the client more comfortable.
2. Arrange for a professional interpreter despite the family's refusal.
3. Use simple English and gestures to communicate with the client.
4. Ignore the language barrier and continue with the treatment.

Answer Key

The correct answer is: 2. Arrange for a professional interpreter despite the family's refusal.

Topic: Advocacy for Client Rights and Needs

When preparing for the NCLEX exam, it's essential to understand the role of the nurse as an advocate for clients. This role involves promoting and protecting the rights, health, and safety of the client.

In this question, the nurse is in a situation where there's a language barrier with a client who is hard of hearing. While the family's offer to translate might come from a good place, it can potentially lead to misinterpretations, and consequently, to errors in the client's care. Furthermore, relying on family members for translation can sometimes compromise the client's right to privacy and confidentiality.

Therefore, the best option is to arrange for a professional interpreter, despite the family's refusal (Option 2). This ensures that information is conveyed accurately and maintains the client's privacy and confidentiality.

Option 1 is not the best choice as family members may not be proficient in medical terminology and might convey inaccurate information. Option 3 is not the best choice as it may not ensure that the client fully understands the information. Option 4 is incorrect as it can lead to serious misunderstandings and is not respectful of the client's rights and needs.

For the NCLEX, remember that as an advocate, the nurse promotes the client's rights, stands up for the client's needs, and ensures that the client is a partner in their care.

Question 7

A nurse is part of a multidisciplinary team caring for a client with a new diagnosis of type 2 diabetes mellitus. What is the most appropriate action for the nurse to take in this team?

1. Discuss the client's prognosis with the physician.
2. Coordinate with the dietitian to plan the client's meals.
3. Leave the patient education to the endocrinologist.
4. Recommend the client to not ask any questions to the pharmacist about medication.

Answer Key

The correct answer is: 2. Coordinate with the dietitian to plan the client's meals.

Topic: Collaboration with a Multi-Disciplinary Team

Collaboration with a multi-disciplinary team is an important aspect of nursing care. This approach ensures that the client benefits from the unique skills and expertise of each team member, and it promotes comprehensive and coordinated care.

In the context of the NCLEX exam, understanding the roles and responsibilities of different team members is key. Each professional brings a unique perspective and set of skills to the table. Nurses, doctors, dietitians, pharmacists, social workers, and more all work together to provide holistic care to the client.

In the given scenario, the most appropriate action for the nurse is to coordinate with the dietitian to plan the client's meals (Option 2). This ensures the client receives a balanced and suitable diet, which is an important part of diabetes management.

Option 1 is less correct because all team members should be aware of the client's condition and prognosis. Option 3 is incorrect because, although the endocrinologist plays a significant role in diabetes management, patient education is also a core aspect of nursing care. Option 4 is incorrect because encouraging the client to ask questions can improve their understanding of the condition and medication regime, promoting adherence and better outcomes.

Remember, as a nurse, your role in a multi-disciplinary team is to communicate effectively with other healthcare professionals and to ensure that care is client-focused, coordinated, and comprehensive.

Question 8

A nurse is taking care of multiple clients during a busy shift. Which of the following actions best demonstrates effective time management?

1. The nurse performs tasks for the most demanding clients first, regardless of the urgency of their needs.
2. The nurse postpones documentation until the end of the shift to have uninterrupted time.
3. The nurse performs tasks as they come up, without any particular order.
4. The nurse prioritizes tasks based on urgency and combines activities for efficiency.

Answer Key
The correct answer is: 4. The nurse prioritizes tasks based on urgency and combines activities for efficiency.

Topic: Effective Time Management in Nursing

Effective time management is critical in nursing as it helps ensure that all patients receive appropriate care in a timely manner, and that tasks are completed efficiently. This includes the ability to prioritize tasks based on urgency and importance, delegating tasks when appropriate, planning and organizing activities, and using downtime effectively.

In the context of the NCLEX exam, understanding the principles of time management in nursing is key. For instance, in the given scenario, the best demonstration of effective time management is prioritizing tasks based on urgency and combining activities for efficiency (Option 4). This is because it ensures that all clients' needs are met based on their importance and urgency, and that tasks are performed in an organized and efficient manner.

Option 1 is incorrect because taking care of the most demanding clients first may not always align with addressing the most urgent needs. Option 2 is incorrect because delaying documentation can lead to missed or inaccurate information. Option 3 is incorrect because this approach lacks organization and efficiency, which can lead to poor patient care and increased stress for the nurse.

Question 9

The nurse is part of a multidisciplinary team and has a disagreement with another team member regarding a client's care plan. Which of the following is the most appropriate action for the nurse to take in this situation?

1. The nurse should ignore the disagreement to maintain peace within the team.
2. The nurse should insist on their point of view because they know what's best for the client.
3. The nurse should gossip about the disagreement with other team members to gain support.
4. The nurse should initiate a respectful conversation with the team member to understand their perspective and find a resolution.

Answer Key

The correct answer is: 4. The nurse should initiate a respectful conversation with the team member to understand their perspective and find a resolution.

Topic: Conflict Management in Healthcare

Conflict management in healthcare is crucial because disagreements can arise in any team setting, and healthcare is no exception. Conflicts, if not managed effectively, can lead to negative consequences such as reduced team cohesion, poor patient outcomes, and increased stress amongst team members.

In the context of the NCLEX exam, understanding the principles of conflict management in healthcare is important. In the given scenario, the best course of action is for the nurse to initiate a respectful conversation with the team member to understand their perspective and find a resolution (Option 4). This is because it promotes open communication, mutual respect, and collaborative problem-solving, which are essential components of effective conflict management.

Options 1, 2, and 3 are not ideal strategies. Ignoring the disagreement (Option 1) can lead to resentment and may negatively impact patient care. Insisting on one's point of view without considering others' perspectives (Option 2) can create hostility and reduce team cooperation. Gossiping about the disagreement (Option 3) can foster a toxic work environment and break down trust within the team.

For the NCLEX exam, it's important to remember that effective conflict management involves open and respectful communication, understanding differing viewpoints, and collaborative problem-solving to reach the best outcomes for the patient.

Question 10

A nurse overhears another nurse discussing specific details about a client's health condition on a personal phone call in a public area of the hospital. What is the most appropriate action for the nurse to take?

1. Ignore the situation since it does not directly involve them.
2. Confront the nurse in a loud voice to ensure that they know the action is wrong.
3. Report the situation to the nurse manager.
4. Share the information overheard with other colleagues to warn them about the nurse's behavior.

Answer Key

The correct answer is: 3. Report the situation to the nurse manager.

Topic: Maintaining Client Confidentiality and Privacy

Client confidentiality and privacy are fundamental ethical and legal obligations in healthcare. They ensure that clients' personal health information is protected and shared only when necessary for their care and treatment. Violating confidentiality can lead to serious consequences, including damage to the nurse-client relationship, potential legal action, and harm to the client's well-being.

In the scenario presented, the nurse overheard a colleague discussing specific client details in a public area, which is a breach of confidentiality. The NCLEX exam tests your ability to handle such ethical dilemmas appropriately.

Option 3, reporting the situation to the nurse manager, is the most suitable action. It allows the situation to be handled in a formal and professional manner, ensuring accountability, remedial action, and the prevention of future breaches.

Option 1, ignoring the situation, is inappropriate because it allows the breach of confidentiality to continue. Option 2, confronting the nurse in a loud voice, is not professional and may exacerbate the situation. Option 4, sharing the overheard information with other colleagues, is another breach of confidentiality and should be avoided.

When preparing for the NCLEX, it's essential to remember the importance of maintaining client confidentiality and privacy and the correct ways to handle any breaches you might encounter.

Question 11

A nurse is preparing to hand off care to the oncoming shift for a client who was admitted with pneumonia. Which of the following information should the nurse include in the report?

1. The client's preference for breakfast items.
2. A brief summary of the client's family history.
3. Changes in the client's oxygen saturation and response to treatment.
4. The friendly chat the nurse had with the client about their hobbies.

Answer Key

The correct answer is: 3. Changes in the client's oxygen saturation and response to treatment.

Topic: Handoff of Care Reporting

Handoff of care reporting is an essential nursing skill, ensuring continuity and safety in patient care. It involves communicating critical patient information to the next healthcare provider when a shift change occurs or the patient transitions to a different care area.

This information typically includes the patient's current condition, recent changes, ongoing treatment, care plan goals, and tasks that need to be completed. It should be concise, relevant, and focused on the patient's immediate care needs.

In the given question, option 3, changes in the client's oxygen saturation and response to treatment, provides relevant, immediate, and important information about the client's current health status, making it the correct answer.

Options 1 and 4, regarding the client's breakfast preferences and hobbies, are non-urgent and non-clinical details. While these are valuable for holistic care and developing rapport, they are not prioritized in a handoff report. Option 2, a brief summary of the client's family history, is generally not necessary in a shift change report unless it directly impacts the client's current condition or care.

To prepare for the NCLEX, remember that effective handoff reporting is crucial for patient safety and effective continuity of care. Practice prioritizing information and presenting it clearly and concisely.

Question 12

A nurse is documenting the care provided to a client who has a wound. Which of the following statements should the nurse include in the documentation?

1. "The wound seems a bit better."
2. "The client felt comfortable with the dressing change."
3. "The wound measures 3 cm in length, 2 cm in width, with pink granulation tissue."
4. "The client is happy with the wound care."

Answer Key

The correct answer is: 3. "The wound measures 3 cm in length, 2 cm in width, with pink granulation tissue."

Topic: Approved Terminology in Documenting Care

When documenting patient care in the medical record, it's essential to use objective, factual, and precise language. This ensures that the documentation is accurate, clear, and professional, providing a reliable basis for patient care decisions and potential legal reference.

In the question presented, option 3 provides the most objective, factual, and specific information about the wound's condition. It includes specific measurements and descriptions, which are part of approved terminology for documenting care.

Option 1 uses vague language ("seems a bit better") and doesn't provide specific, measurable details about the wound's progress. Option 2 and 4 focus on the patient's feelings, which, while important, are not as crucial as objective assessments when documenting wound care.

Preparing for the NCLEX exam, it's important to focus on using accurate, specific, and approved medical terminology in all areas of nursing practice, including documentation. Ensure you are familiar with common terms and abbreviations used in your field and are comfortable with using them appropriately. Always remember to focus on objective and

49

measurable observations rather than subjective descriptions or assumptions.

Question 13

The nurse is preparing to transfer a client from the medical-surgical unit to the intensive care unit (ICU). Which of the following steps should the nurse prioritize to ensure a safe transfer?

1. Inform the client and the family about the new room location.
2. Prepare the client's belongings for the move.
3. Review and communicate the client's current status, recent changes, and plan of care with the receiving nurse.
4. Ensure the client's meal is served before the transfer.

Answer Key
The correct answer is: 3. Review and communicate the client's current status, recent changes, and plan of care with the receiving nurse.

Topic: Safe Admission, Transfer, and Discharge Procedures

When preparing for the NCLEX, it's important to understand the procedures and responsibilities involved in the safe transfer of clients between different units or facilities. Ensuring a smooth, safe transition involves multiple steps, among which effective communication of the client's current status and plan of care to the receiving healthcare provider is a priority.

In the provided question, option 3 is the most critical step to ensure safe transfer. This step allows for continuity of care and reduces the risk of errors or misunderstandings. The information provided should be accurate, up-to-date, and complete, including relevant medical history, current health status, any recent changes, ongoing treatments, and any other significant data related to the client's care.

While informing the client and family (option 1), preparing the client's belongings for the move (option 2), and ensuring the client has eaten (option 4) are all important steps in the transfer process, they do not directly impact the continuity and safety of the client's medical care.

During your NCLEX preparation, make sure you familiarize yourself with all aspects of safe client transfer, including effective communication strategies, documentation requirements, and potential challenges to avoid. Always remember that the client's health and safety are the top priorities during any transfer or discharge process.

Question 14

The nurse in a medical-surgical unit is assigned to care for four clients. In which order should the nurse prioritize care for these clients?

1. A client who was recently diagnosed with diabetes and needs education on blood glucose monitoring.
2. A client with a deep vein thrombosis reporting sudden onset of chest pain and shortness of breath.
3. A client with hypertension who is due for their daily blood pressure medication.
4. A client scheduled for a chest X-ray in 2 hours.

Answer Key
The correct order is: 2, 3, 1, 4.

Topic: Prioritizing Care Based on Acuity

A key skill for nursing professionals is the ability to prioritize care based on acuity levels of patients. The NCLEX examination will often present scenarios where you must identify the most critical or urgent situation to address.

In the above question, prioritizing care should be based on the urgency of the situation and potential risk to the patient's life.

The client with a deep vein thrombosis reporting sudden onset of chest pain and shortness of breath (option 2) could be experiencing a life-threatening pulmonary embolism and should be attended to immediately.

The client with hypertension who is due for their daily blood pressure medication (option 3) should be next, as maintaining blood pressure levels is essential for preventing complications.

The newly diagnosed diabetic patient (option 1) requires education on managing their condition, but this is not as immediately urgent as the situations in options 2 and 3.

Lastly, the client scheduled for a chest X-ray in 2 hours (option 4) is least urgent as this procedure is scheduled and does not require immediate action.

When studying for the NCLEX, remember the principles of prioritizing: address life-threatening situations first, then urgent but not life-threatening needs, followed by important but non-urgent needs. Understanding these principles will help you make appropriate decisions in the complex, fast-paced environment of healthcare.

Question 15

A nurse encounters a situation where a client with terminal cancer has requested not to be resuscitated, but the client's family insists on full resuscitative measures. How should the nurse handle this situation?

1. Respect the client's wishes and do not resuscitate.
2. Respect the family's wishes and perform resuscitation.
3. Seek guidance from the hospital's ethics committee.
4. Inform the family that it is the client's decision and they have no say in the matter.

Answer Key
The correct answer is: 3.

Topic: Ethical Dilemmas in Nursing

Ethical dilemmas are common in healthcare and can often present complex challenges. When faced with an ethical dilemma, it's crucial for nurses to understand the ethical principles of autonomy, beneficence, nonmaleficence, justice, and fidelity.

In the above question, the client's wish for a 'Do Not Resuscitate' (DNR) order conflicts with the family's desire for full resuscitative measures. This situation represents a clash between the ethical principle of autonomy (respecting the client's right to make decisions about their own health care) and the principle of beneficence (taking actions to benefit others, in this case, the family's wish to prolong the client's life).

The best option in such a scenario (option 3) is to seek guidance from the hospital's ethics committee, a group of individuals who are trained to help navigate such ethical dilemmas. They can facilitate discussions between the healthcare team, the client, and the family, with the goal of reaching a resolution that respects the client's wishes and considers the family's concerns.

Question 16

A nurse witnesses a colleague taking extra supplies home from the hospital. Which action by the nurse aligns best with the Nurses' Code of Ethics?

1. Ignore the situation as it does not directly impact patient care.
2. Confront the colleague directly and demand they return the supplies.
3. Report the incident to a supervisor.
4. Discuss the incident with other colleagues to see if they have noticed similar behavior.

Answer Key

The correct answer is: 3.

Topic: Nurses' Code of Ethics

The Nurses' Code of Ethics is a guide for carrying out nursing responsibilities in a manner consistent with quality in nursing care and the ethical obligations of the profession. One of the key provisions in the code is the responsibility to maintain integrity in the profession.

In the scenario provided, the nurse is witnessing a colleague behaving unethically by taking supplies from the hospital, which constitutes theft and can impact hospital resources and, indirectly, patient care. Ignoring the situation (option 1) or discussing it with other colleagues (option 4) would not be appropriate actions and could contribute to a culture of unethical behavior.

Direct confrontation (option 2) may be confrontational and could potentially escalate the situation without a resolution. The best choice here is for the nurse to report the incident to a supervisor (option 3). This action aligns with the ethical responsibility of maintaining integrity in the profession, ensuring that concerns are addressed through proper channels, and promoting an ethical workplace.

Question 17

A nurse is preparing to administer a new medication to a client. Which of the following actions should the nurse take to ensure informed consent for care?

1. Ask the client if they have any allergies.
2. Tell the client that the medication is safe they likely will not experience side effects.
3. Provide the client with information about the purpose of the medication, how it works, potential side effects, and alternatives.
4. Administer the medication as soon as possible to ensure the client's health.

Answer Key
The correct answer is: 3.

Topic: Client Education and Consent for Care

Informed consent is a critical aspect of providing care. It is based on the principle of respect for autonomy, which means that individuals have the right to make decisions about their own healthcare. To give informed consent, clients must have enough information to make an informed decision about whether to accept or refuse treatment.

For informed consent to be valid, it must be voluntary (the decision is made freely without coercion), informed (the person has been given enough information to make an educated decision), and the person must have the capacity to make the decision (they understand the information provided and can weigh the risks and benefits).

When administering a new medication, the nurse should provide the client with comprehensive information about the medication. This includes explaining the purpose of the medication, how it works, potential side effects, and alternatives (option 3). Simply asking about allergies (option 1) is not sufficient for informed consent. Telling the client that the medication has no side effects (option 2) is misleading and does not give a full picture of potential risks.

Administering the medication as quickly as possible (option 4) without providing the necessary information does not respect the client's autonomy.

By giving comprehensive information about the treatment, the nurse ensures the client can make an informed decision about their care, respecting their rights and upholding ethical standards. This approach to client education and consent is crucial for nurses to understand as they prepare for the NCLEX exam.

Question 18

The nurse is reading a healthcare provider's new orders for a client with heart failure. The order includes starting the client on a new medication. Which of the following is the correct sequence of actions the nurse should take in implementing this order?

1. Check the client's medical record for any drug allergies, administer the medication, and then document the administration.
2. Administer the medication, check the client's response to the medication, and then document the administration.
3. Verify the medication order with another nurse, check the client's medical record for any drug allergies, administer the medication, and then document the administration.
4. Document the medication administration, administer the medication, and then verify the order with the healthcare provider.

Answer Key
The correct answer is: 3.

Topic: Implementation of Healthcare Provider Orders

Implementing healthcare provider orders is a significant role of the nurse and requires careful consideration to ensure patient safety and effective treatment. When implementing a new medication order, the nurse should first verify the medication order for accuracy (option 3). This often includes checking it against the original order and consulting with another healthcare professional as necessary. It's an essential step in preventing medication errors and ensuring the order is correct.

Next, the nurse should check the client's medical record for any drug allergies. This is to ensure that the client does not have a known allergy to the new medication, which could cause an adverse reaction.

Following verification of the order and checking for allergies, the nurse can safely administer the medication. After administration, the nurse must then document the medication administration in the client's medical record, noting the time, dosage, route, and any immediate observable effects.

While all the options listed involve elements of medication administration, only option 3 correctly orders the steps in the process. Administering the medication before checking for allergies (options 1 and 2) could be dangerous, and documenting administration before it has occurred (option 4) is not accurate record-keeping.

Question 19

A nurse on a busy medical-surgical unit is caring for multiple clients with complex needs. In planning for quality client care, the nurse should utilize which of the following resources? Select all that apply.

1. Pharmacy consultation for medication questions.
2. Social worker involvement for discharge planning.
3. Physical therapy assessment for mobility issues.
4. Personal judgement and experience to adjust medication dosages.
5. Dietary services for a client with nutritional needs.

Answer Key
The correct answers are: 1, 2, 3, and 5.

Topic: Utilizing Resources for Quality Client Care

Effective utilization of resources is a crucial skill in nursing to provide quality client care. In a complex healthcare setting, a nurse often has to collaborate with other professionals from different disciplines to address the diverse needs of the clients. This multidisciplinary approach ensures that clients receive comprehensive care that addresses all aspects of their health.

Pharmacy consultation (option 1) can provide valuable information about medications, such as dosages, administration times, potential side effects, and interactions. Pharmacists have specialized knowledge in this area and can assist in optimizing medication regimens for clients.

Social workers (option 2) play an essential role in discharge planning, addressing social determinants of health, and connecting clients with community resources. They can help to ensure a smooth transition from hospital to home or another care setting.

Physical therapists (option 3) can assess and treat mobility issues, helping clients to improve their strength, balance, and overall function. They can devise personalized therapy programs and provide education on safe mobility practices.

Adjusting medication dosages based on personal judgement (option 4) is not within the scope of nursing practice. Medication orders should only be changed by a healthcare provider, and any concerns about medications should be communicated to the appropriate person.

Dietary services (option 5) can address clients' nutritional needs by providing tailored meal plans, dietary advice, and nutritional supplements. They can also collaborate with the healthcare team to manage conditions such as diabetes or malnutrition.

Question 20

A newly hired nurse is assigned to care for a client who requires a complex wound dressing change, which she has never performed before. Which of the following is the most appropriate action for the nurse to take?

1. Attempt the procedure, relying on her fundamental nursing knowledge.
2. Ask a colleague to do the dressing change while she watches.
3. Look up the procedure in the nursing procedures manual and then perform it.
4. Inform the charge nurse about her limitation and ask for supervision or training.

Answer Key
The correct answer is 4.

Topic: Recognizing and Reporting Limitations of Self and Others

Recognizing and reporting limitations of self and others is a vital aspect of nursing practice. This ensures patient safety, maintains the quality of care, and supports continuous learning and professional growth.

Attempting to perform a procedure without the necessary experience or skillset (option 1) is risky and can lead to potential harm to the client. It also violates the nursing standard of practice that calls for competence in all nursing interventions.

While observing a colleague perform the procedure (option 2) or referring to a procedures manual (option 3) may be helpful for learning, it is not an adequate replacement for proper training or supervision, particularly for complex or high-risk procedures.

The most appropriate action in this scenario is for the nurse to inform the charge nurse of her limitation and request supervision or training (option 4). This demonstrates professional responsibility, self-awareness, and a commitment to client safety.

As you prepare for the NCLEX, remember that recognizing your limitations and asking for help when necessary is not a sign of weakness, but rather a hallmark of safe and effective nursing practice. Understanding your scope of practice, continually improving your skills through education and training, and advocating for patient safety are critical aspects of successful nursing practice.

Question 21

The nurse is providing care for a client who has multiple injuries due to domestic violence. Which of the following actions should the nurse take according to the legal obligations?

1. Encourage the client to report the abuse to the police.
2. Document the client's injuries and report them to the charge nurse.
3. Keep the information confidential as the client requests not to disclose it.
4. Document the client's injuries and report the situation to the appropriate authorities.

Answer Key

The correct answer is 4.

Topic: Reporting Client Conditions as Required by Law

Reporting client conditions as required by law is a key aspect of the nurse's role, especially when it comes to issues such as child abuse, elder abuse, and domestic violence. In many jurisdictions, healthcare providers are legally obligated to report suspected or known cases of abuse, regardless of the victim's wishes.

Encouraging the client to report the abuse to the police (option 1) is not enough as the nurse has a legal and ethical obligation to report the situation.

Documenting the client's injuries and reporting them to the charge nurse (option 2) is part of the nurse's role, but it does not fulfill the legal requirement for reporting to appropriate authorities.

Keeping the information confidential because the client requests it (option 3) is not applicable in this case. Despite the importance of client confidentiality, laws requiring the reporting of domestic violence take precedence.

The correct action is to document the client's injuries and report the situation to the appropriate authorities (option 4). This fulfills the nurse's legal obligation, protects the client, and may help initiate the provision of further support services.

Question 22

The nurse is preparing to administer a medication to a client. The medication was prescribed by a healthcare provider who is not part of the hospital's medical staff. What should the nurse do?

1. Administer the medication as ordered.
2. Confirm the order with the charge nurse before administering the medication.
3. Contact the prescribing provider for more information about the order.
4. Refuse to administer the medication until it is prescribed by a provider who is part of the hospital's medical staff.

Answer Key
The correct answer is 4.

Topic: Legal Scope of Nursing Practice

The legal scope of nursing practice often includes the administration of medications. However, this does not mean that nurses can administer any medication ordered by any provider. Nurses must ensure that the medication orders they follow are given by a healthcare provider who has the authority to prescribe medications within the specific healthcare facility.

Option 1 is incorrect because, even though the provider may be licensed to prescribe medication, they may not have the authority to prescribe in the particular hospital where the nurse is working.

Option 2 is not enough because the charge nurse does not have the power to authorize a medication order given by a provider who does not have privileges at the hospital.

Option 3 is incorrect because calling the provider for more information will not change the fact that they are not authorized to prescribe at the hospital.

Option 4 is correct. Nurses must know the policies of their specific healthcare facility and adhere to them. This means refusing to administer medications ordered by providers who are not part of the hospital's medical staff.

When studying for the NCLEX, remember the importance of understanding the legal scope of nursing practice. This includes knowing who can provide medication orders, under what circumstances, and within what settings. It also requires the nurse to understand their role in verifying orders and refusing those that fall outside legal or institutional guidelines.

Question 23

The nurse is assigned to participate in a performance improvement project focused on reducing the incidence of hospital-acquired infections (HAIs). Which of the following actions would be most beneficial for the nurse to take first in this project?

1. Implement new hand hygiene protocols immediately.
2. Conduct an education session on infection control for all staff.
3. Review the current literature on evidence-based practices for reducing HAIs.
4. Discourage visitors to the hospital to limit potential sources of infection.

Answer Key
The correct answer is 3.

Topic: Participation in Performance Improvement Projects

Performance improvement projects in healthcare settings are often directed towards improving patient outcomes, such as reducing the incidence of HAIs. These projects should be data-driven and based on the best available evidence.

Option 1 is incorrect as implementing new protocols immediately, without examining the current situation or reviewing the best evidence, may not lead to the desired outcomes and could potentially create new problems.

Option 2 might be a part of the project but conducting an education session before understanding the evidence and identifying the specific needs in the hospital would be premature.

Option 3 is the best initial step. Reviewing the current literature on evidence-based practices for reducing HAIs can provide a foundation for the project. It can help to identify proven strategies, learn from the experiences of others, and guide the project's direction.

Option 4 is not an effective strategy. Limiting visitors can have negative impacts on patient wellbeing and may not significantly reduce the risk of HAIs.

Question 24

A nurse is caring for a client who has just been diagnosed with type 2 diabetes. The client appears overwhelmed and anxious. Which of the following actions should the nurse take first in this situation?

1. Refer the client to a dietitian for nutrition counseling.
2. Refer the client to a psychologist for emotional support.
3. Refer the client to a diabetes educator for diabetes management training.
4. Arrange for a home health nurse to visit the client at home.

Answer Key
The correct answer is 3.

Topic: Assessing the Need for Referrals

When a client is newly diagnosed with a chronic condition like type 2 diabetes, it is crucial to assess the client's needs and refer appropriately to help manage the condition effectively. The nurse, as an integral part of the healthcare team, plays a vital role in recognizing when clients require additional services and making suitable referrals.

Option 1 is important as diet plays a significant role in diabetes management, but it's not the first step. Option 2 might be necessary later, particularly if the client continues to feel overwhelmed and anxious despite receiving education and support. Option 4 can be useful for clients who require assistance with self-care activities at home.

However, option 3 is the most appropriate first step. A diabetes educator can provide comprehensive education on blood sugar monitoring, medication administration, dietary modifications, and lifestyle changes. This knowledge is essential for the client to manage their condition effectively and reduce the risk of complications.

In preparation for the NCLEX, remember that effective referral is an important aspect of nursing practice. Nurses should prioritize referrals based on the client's immediate needs and the potential impact on their health and wellbeing.

Question 25

A nurse is caring for a client who has a known peanut allergy. Which of the following actions is most important for the nurse to take during the client's hospital stay?

1. Educating the client to avoid any food products containing peanuts.
2. Ensuring the client wears an allergy identification band.
3. Providing the client with a menu free of peanut products.
4. Ensuring epinephrine is readily available.

Answer Key

The correct answer is 2.

Topic: Allergy Assessment and Intervention

In the setting of a healthcare facility, it is crucial to ensure that the entire healthcare team is aware of the patient's allergies. This information should be prominently displayed in the patient's health record and visibly indicated, typically by an allergy identification band. This will alert all caregivers and healthcare workers about the allergy and help prevent accidental exposure to the allergen.

Option 1 is certainly important, and client education forms an integral part of care. However, in the context of a hospital stay, it's essential to prioritize strategies that involve the entire healthcare team.

Option 3 is also significant, but a client may receive food from outside sources, not just the hospital's food service.

Option 4 is important in case of an allergic reaction. Still, the primary goal should be to prevent an allergic reaction from occurring in the first place.

When preparing for the NCLEX, remember that the goal of allergy management is prevention. By correctly identifying and alerting the entire healthcare team to the allergy, nurses play a pivotal role in preventing allergic reactions and ensuring the safety of their clients.

Question 26

The nurse is preparing to admit a client who is being treated for bacterial meningitis. In which type of room should the nurse plan to place the client?

1. A private room.
2. A room with another client who is also being treated for bacterial meningitis.
3. A room with a client who has a respiratory infection.
4. A semi-private room.

Answer Key
The correct answer is 1.

Topic: Client Care Environment Assessment

Bacterial meningitis is a highly contagious disease that is often spread through respiratory droplets. To protect other clients, those with bacterial meningitis should be placed in a private room under droplet precautions.

Option 2 is not advisable because even if both clients are being treated for bacterial meningitis, they could potentially have different strains of the bacteria which could complicate their treatment.

Option 3 is not advisable as the client with the respiratory infection is likely already immunocompromised and at a higher risk for contracting other illnesses.

Option 4 is not advisable as it could put the other client in the semi-private room at risk.

In preparation for the NCLEX, understanding the types of isolation and when to use them is crucial. Isolation precautions are based on the mode of transmission of the disease. These measures help to control the spread of illnesses and protect both the patient and the healthcare worker. In this case, the client with bacterial meningitis should be placed in a private room with droplet precautions implemented.

Question 27

A nurse is working on a unit that is short-staffed and there is an increased number of clients. Which of the following actions should the nurse take to ensure staff safety?

1. Ask staff to skip breaks to accommodate the increased workload.
2. Request assistance from other units or float nurses.
3. Encourage staff to work faster to meet client needs.
4. Inform clients that care may be delayed due to understaffing.

Answer Key

The correct answer is 2.

Topic: Promoting Staff Safety

Staff safety is critical in a healthcare setting. When the workload increases due to a higher number of clients, the best approach is to request additional help. This might mean getting assistance from other units or calling in float nurses. This maintains the staff-to-client ratio and ensures that all clients receive the necessary care without overworking the current staff.

Option 1 is not a good choice, as skipping breaks can lead to fatigue and increase the risk of errors, affecting both staff safety and patient care.

Option 3 is also not advisable because rushing can lead to mistakes and potential harm to clients and staff.

Option 4 may be a last resort, but it should not be the first action taken. Communication with clients about delays is important, but the primary action should be to ensure adequate staffing to meet the increased demand.

In preparation for the NCLEX, it's important to understand that promoting safety for healthcare staff is just as crucial as promoting safety for clients. Safe staffing levels reduce the risk of staff fatigue, burnout, and errors in client care. Always advocate for safe work conditions and adequate staffing levels.

Question 28

A nurse is planning an education session for a group of older adults living in a retirement community. Which of the following topics should the nurse include in order to best promote client injury prevention?

1. The importance of annual flu vaccinations.
2. Strategies for managing chronic illnesses.
3. Ways to prevent slips, trips, and falls in the home.
4. Methods to improve memory and cognition.

Answer Key
The correct answer is 3.

Topic: Client Injury Prevention

Injury prevention is a key aspect of nursing care, particularly for older adults who may be at a higher risk due to factors such as decreased mobility, poor balance, and impaired vision. Falls are a leading cause of injury in older adults, so educating this population about ways to prevent slips, trips, and falls in the home is a critical part of injury prevention.

Strategies can include simple actions such as clearing walkways, securing loose rugs, installing handrails in bathrooms, using non-slip mats, and improving lighting. Encourage older adults to use assistive devices as needed, to maintain regular physical activity to improve strength and balance, and to have regular vision checks.

While options 1, 2, and 4 are important health topics for older adults, they do not directly address injury prevention.

Question 29

A nurse is preparing to administer medication to a hospitalized client. Which of the following actions is the most appropriate way for the nurse to ensure the correct client identification?

1. Check the client's room number.
2. Ask the client to confirm their full name and birthdate.
3. Look at the client's picture on the electronic health record.
4. Call the client by name and proceed if they respond.

Answer Key
The correct answer is 2.

Topic: Client Identification Procedures

Client identification is a critical step in delivering safe and effective care. It helps to prevent errors such as administering medication to the wrong client. According to the Joint Commission's National Patient Safety Goals, at least two patient identifiers should be used when providing care, treatment, and services. These identifiers can include the client's name, an assigned identification number, telephone number, or birth date.

Relying solely on room numbers or physical appearance can lead to errors, especially in settings where clients might be moved or discharged frequently. While checking a photo ID can be useful, it should not be the only method of identification. Asking the client to state their full name and birth date ensures that the client is actively involved in the identification process, enhancing the safety and accuracy of care.

For the NCLEX, it is essential to understand the importance of using multiple, reliable methods for client identification and involving the client in this process whenever possible. Patient safety is a key aspect of nursing practice and a major area of focus on the exam.

Question 30

A nurse receives a written medication order from a healthcare provider that reads: "Digoxin 0.25 mg PO daily." Which of the following actions should the nurse take next?

1. Administer the medication to the client immediately.
2. Call the pharmacy and ask for the medication.
3. Verify the appropriateness of the order with the healthcare provider.
4. Document the order in the client's medication administration record.

Answer Key
The correct answer is 3.

Topic: Verification of Treatment Order Appropriateness

Before implementing any treatment orders, it's crucial that the nurse verifies the appropriateness of the order based on the client's current condition, the nurse's knowledge, and established standards of care. For instance, in the case of Digoxin, it's necessary to consider the client's heart rate, potassium levels, renal function, and other medications.

In some cases, it may be necessary to clarify or verify an order with the healthcare provider before carrying it out. This could be due to a variety of reasons including uncertainty about the order, a perceived error, or simply the need for more information.

On the NCLEX, understanding this process is key because it falls under the nurse's scope of practice to ensure that all treatment orders are suitable for the client's current state. Nurses play a pivotal role in promoting client safety, which includes questioning and verifying orders when necessary.

Question 31

During an emergency preparedness drill, a nurse is assigned to the triage area. Which client should the nurse identify as the highest priority to receive treatment?

1. A client with a compound fracture of the leg, who is alert and oriented.
2. A client who has chest pain and is short of breath.
3. A client who is unconscious, with shallow and irregular respirations.
4. A client with an abrasion on the forehead, who is awake and talking.

Answer Key
The correct answer is 3.

Topic: Emergency Planning and Response

Emergency Planning and Response is a critical topic in nursing and can appear in different contexts on the NCLEX. Nurses play a significant role in managing healthcare emergencies, both within the healthcare setting and at the community level.

At its core, emergency response planning involves preparing for unexpected events or disasters, which may be natural (like earthquakes or hurricanes) or man-made (like a chemical spill or act of terrorism). These situations often involve dealing with multiple casualties, making it necessary to prioritize who gets treated first. This is where the concept of triage comes into play.

Triage is the process of determining the priority of patients' treatments based on the severity of their condition. The goal is to do the greatest good for the greatest number of patients. In a mass casualty situation, priority is typically given to those patients who have a critical need for treatment and a reasonable chance of survival if they receive timely care.

In the context of the given question, the unconscious client with shallow and irregular respirations (option 3) should be identified as the highest priority. This client exhibits signs of severe respiratory distress, a life-threatening condition. They require immediate intervention to secure their airway and stabilize their breathing.

The chest pain and shortness of breath (option 2) could indicate a heart condition, which also requires prompt attention but is less immediately life-threatening than a compromised airway. The compound fracture (option 1) is a serious injury but does not present an immediate threat to life. The client with the abrasion on the forehead (option 4) has a minor injury in comparison to the others and can be treated later.

Preparing for the NCLEX requires a deep understanding of the principles of triage and emergency response. Questions on this topic test your ability to make quick and accurate assessments of patient conditions and prioritize care under pressure. Remember, in emergency situations, saving lives and reducing suffering are the primary goals. This often means prioritizing care based on acuity, not on a first-come, first-serve basis.

Question 32

A nurse is caring for a client who needs to be moved from the bed to a wheelchair. Which of the following actions by the nurse is an example of utilizing ergonomic principles?

1. The nurse enlists the help of a colleague to move the client.
2. The nurse encourages the client to do as much as possible independently.
3. The nurse uses a transfer belt when moving the client.
4. All of the above.

Answer Key
The correct answer is 4.

Topic: Using Ergonomic Principles in Care

Ergonomics in nursing involves applying scientific information concerning humans to the design of objects, systems, and environment for human use. In the context of healthcare, it primarily refers to promoting safety and preventing injury (both for patients and healthcare workers) through the design and modification of work environments and processes.

When it comes to patient handling tasks such as transfers, lifts, and repositioning, using ergonomic principles can significantly reduce the risk of injury. Musculoskeletal disorders are common among healthcare workers due to the physical demands of their job, and proper ergonomics can help prevent these injuries.

In the context of the question, all the options provided demonstrate the use of ergonomic principles:

1. Enlisting the help of a colleague can reduce the physical strain on one person and help ensure the safety of both the client and the nurse (option 1).
2. Encouraging the client to do as much as possible independently can reduce the need for physical exertion from the nurse and also empower the client (option 2).

3. Using a transfer belt can reduce the risk of falls and injuries by providing a secure and safe grip during transfers (option 3).

Therefore, the correct answer is "All of the above" (option 4).

Preparing for the NCLEX requires a deep understanding of the principles of ergonomics and how they can be applied in patient care. Questions on this topic test your ability to make informed decisions about patient handling tasks that promote safety and prevent injury. Remember, the health and safety of both the client and the healthcare provider are paramount, and understanding how to apply ergonomic principles in care is key to ensuring this.

Question 33

A nurse is teaching a new healthcare worker about proper handling of biohazardous materials. Which of the following information should the nurse include in the teaching?

1. Use standard precautions for all clients, regardless of their infection status.
2. Dispose of biohazardous waste in a regular trash bin.
3. Reuse needles and sharps if they look clean.
4. It is not necessary to wear gloves when handling body fluids if they don't contain visible blood.

Answer Key
The correct answer is 1.

Topic: Handling Biohazardous and Hazardous Materials

When handling biohazardous and hazardous materials, it's essential to maintain a high standard of safety and hygiene. These materials can include sharps, blood, body fluids, and other substances that may contain pathogens. Improper handling can lead to the transmission of infections and diseases.

The correct choice, option 1, refers to the "Standard Precautions" - guidelines developed by the CDC to reduce the risk of transmission of bloodborne and other pathogens in hospitals. They apply to all patients, regardless of suspected or confirmed infection status, in any setting where healthcare is delivered.

The other options contain incorrect information:
1. Option 2 is incorrect. Biohazardous waste should never be disposed of in a regular trash bin. It must be put into a designated, clearly labeled biohazardous waste container.
2. Option 3 is wrong. Needles and sharps should never be reused, even if they look clean. This can risk transmission of infectious diseases.
3. Option 4 is also incorrect. It is always necessary to wear appropriate personal protective equipment, like

gloves, when handling body fluids, even if there's no visible blood. You can't always see or know if pathogens are present.

For the NCLEX, understanding the protocols for handling biohazardous and hazardous materials is critical. Nurses are on the front line of preventing the spread of infections, so make sure to review these guidelines carefully as part of your study plan.

Question 34

A nurse is providing safety education to a client who is being discharged after hip replacement surgery. Which of the following statements made by the client indicates a need for further teaching?

1. "I will install grab bars in the bathroom."
2. "I will use a reacher to pick up items from the floor."
3. "I will climb stairs multiple times a day to build strength."
4. "I will arrange for help with tasks like cooking and cleaning."

Answer Key
The correct answer is 3.

Topic: Client Safety Education

Client safety education is a crucial part of nursing care. As a nurse, your goal is to provide clients with the knowledge they need to avoid injuries and take an active role in their healthcare.

In the given scenario, the client who underwent a hip replacement surgery has to take care of his new hip and avoid activities that could lead to injury or complications. The client's statement in option 3 indicates a misunderstanding about post-operative care after hip replacement surgery. Climbing stairs multiple times a day, especially in the early stages of recovery, could put too much stress on the new hip and lead to injury or complications. It is recommended to limit stair climbing to once or twice a day in the first weeks following surgery.

Option 1 is correct; installing grab bars in the bathroom can prevent falls. Option 2 is also correct; using a reacher can help the client avoid bending or stretching excessively. Option 4 is correct as well; having assistance for tasks can prevent falls and other accidents while the client is recovering.

This question type is common on the NCLEX. Always pay attention to what the client says, as it can indicate their level of understanding about their care. Your role as a nurse is to correct any misconceptions and provide the most accurate and relevant information to ensure the client's safety and wellbeing.

Question 35

A nurse accidentally gives a patient a double dose of medication due to a misread medication order. What is the most appropriate initial action for the nurse to take?

1. Document the error in the patient's medical record and notify the physician.
2. Document the error on an incident report form and not mention it in the patient's medical record.
3. Inform the patient about the error, document the error on an incident report form, and notify the physician.
4. Tell the charge nurse about the error but avoid mentioning it in the patient's medical record or on an incident report form.

Answer Key
The correct answer is 3.

Topic: Documenting Practice Errors and Near Misses

Documenting practice errors and near misses is a critical aspect of maintaining safety and quality in healthcare settings. Nurses have a professional and ethical responsibility to report errors and near misses. Doing so allows healthcare teams to understand what went wrong and take steps to prevent similar errors in the future.

In the given scenario, the nurse should first ensure the safety of the patient and then carry out three actions: notify the patient about the error (as patients have a right to know about the care they receive), document the error in an incident report form, and notify the physician for potential intervention.

Option 1 and 2 are not entirely correct as both neglect the need to inform the patient. Option 4 is incorrect as it lacks any formal documentation of the error. Remember, when documenting errors or near misses, the aim is not to blame individuals but to understand the underlying systems and processes that contributed to the error.

Question 36

A nurse observes a fellow nurse colleague not adhering to proper hand hygiene protocols prior to administering medications to a client. What should be the first step in addressing this issue?

1. Inform the nurse manager immediately.
2. Talk to the colleague privately about the observed behavior.
3. Report the colleague to the state nursing board.
4. Ignore the situation, as it is not the nurse's responsibility.

Answer Key
The correct answer is 2.

Topic: Reporting Unsafe Practice of Healthcare Personnel

The process of reporting unsafe practices among healthcare personnel is an integral part of maintaining safety and quality in healthcare. In situations where a nurse observes a colleague engaging in unsafe practices, it's crucial to address the issue effectively and professionally.

The first step should ideally be addressing the concern with the colleague directly and privately, as this can often resolve the situation without escalating it further. This action reflects option 2 and is the most appropriate response. It's essential to approach this conversation with a focus on patient safety rather than personal accusation.

Option 1, reporting the concern to the nurse manager, might be a subsequent step if the colleague doesn't respond to direct feedback or if the behavior continues. However, it isn't the first choice because it is always better to try to solve the issue at the lowest level possible.

Option 3 is excessive for this situation and might be appropriate for situations involving severe negligence or misconduct. Option 4 is incorrect, as all healthcare workers have a responsibility to ensure patient safety.

For the NCLEX examination, understanding how to handle scenarios of unsafe practices is important. Questions may ask about the best initial response, requiring you to recognize the most effective and professional way to manage the situation. Always consider the steps that prioritize patient safety, effective communication, and professional ethics.

Question 37

A newly hired nurse is about to use a piece of equipment she is not familiar with for a client procedure. What should be the nurse's best course of action?

1. Proceed to use the equipment, following the manufacturer's instructions.
2. Ask a fellow nurse to guide her on how to use the equipment.
3. Request that a more experienced nurse perform the procedure instead.
4. Postpone the procedure until she has received training on the equipment.

Answer Key
The correct answer is 4.

Topic: Safe Use of Equipment

The safe use of equipment in nursing care is crucial in promoting patient safety and ensuring quality care. Nurses must be well-trained and confident in their ability to use all types of medical equipment to provide the necessary care.

In the given situation, the nurse is unfamiliar with a piece of equipment required for a client procedure. The most appropriate action for the nurse to take is to postpone the procedure until she has received training on the equipment (option 4). Patient safety should always be the top priority, and using equipment without proper training can put the patient at risk.

Option 1 is not advisable as solely relying on the manufacturer's instructions without hands-on training can still lead to misuse or error. Similarly, option 2 may not be sufficient as it doesn't ensure that the nurse has enough understanding and skill to use the equipment safely and effectively in the future.

Option 3 can be a temporary solution, but it does not promote the growth and development of the nurse in question. Nurses must continually update their skills and knowledge about different equipment and their proper usage.

Question 38

A hospital is implementing a new security plan. The nurse manager should ensure that the nursing staff:

1. Read the security plan and sign an agreement.
2. Have access to the security plan and are familiar with the procedures.
3. Only learn about security procedures applicable to their work area.
4. Are given a brief overview of the security plan.

Answer Key
The correct answer is 2.

Topic: Implementing Security Plans and Procedures

Security in healthcare settings is an increasingly important consideration. Effective security plans and procedures protect patients, staff, and property. As such, it is imperative that all staff members, including nursing staff, are not only aware of but also familiar with these procedures.

The nurse manager, in this context, should ensure that nursing staff have access to the security plan and are familiar with the procedures (option 2). This means that the staff should not just be provided with the security plan, but they should understand what the procedures entail and how they should respond in various situations that may arise in their work environment.

Option 1 misses the point of ensuring familiarity with the procedures. Simply reading and signing an agreement doesn't ensure that the staff fully understand or remember all aspects of the security plan.

Option 3 limits the scope of knowledge of the staff, potentially leaving them unprepared for situations outside of their immediate work area. A comprehensive understanding of the security plan and procedures helps ensure a consistent response across the entire facility.

Option 4, a brief overview, is not sufficient as it may not provide in-depth knowledge or understanding needed to respond appropriately in different situations.

When preparing for NCLEX, you should understand the importance of comprehensive knowledge of security plans and procedures. Effective implementation can only occur when all staff members understand the procedures and their roles within them.

Question 39

A newly admitted patient has been diagnosed with Tuberculosis (TB). Which of the following infection prevention principles should the nurse implement?

1. Place the patient in a room with negative pressure ventilation.
2. Encourage the patient to mingle with other patients to improve morale.
3. Administer antibiotics to all other patients in the same unit as a preventative measure.
4. Use standard precautions when caring for the patient.

Answer Key
The correct answer is 1.

Topic: Infection Prevention Principles

Infection prevention is a crucial component of nursing care and is vital in preventing the spread of infectious diseases such as Tuberculosis (TB).

The most appropriate action in this scenario would be to place the patient in a room with negative pressure ventilation (option 1). Negative pressure rooms are used to prevent cross-contamination from room to room. It works by allowing air to flow into the isolation room but not escape from the room, as the air will naturally flow to areas with lower pressure.

Option 2 is incorrect because TB is an airborne disease, which means it can spread to other people in close contact. Encouraging the patient to mingle with others could risk spreading the infection.

Administering antibiotics to all other patients as a preventive measure (option 3) is not an appropriate action. This can lead to unnecessary exposure to antibiotics, risk of allergies, and may contribute to antibiotic resistance.

Option 4, while important, does not fully address the specific precautions needed for a patient with TB. For diseases transmitted by airborne routes such as TB, more than just standard precautions are required.

Question 40

A nurse is educating a group of parents about preventing the spread of common infectious diseases in children. Which of the following instructions would be most appropriate for the nurse to include?

1. Encourage children to share personal items like toothbrushes and towels to promote sharing habits.
2. Advise parents to avoid vaccination as it can cause other illnesses.
3. Teach children to wash their hands before meals and after using the bathroom.
4. Suggest that children should stay home from school only if they are feeling extremely unwell.

Answer Key

The correct answer is 3.

Topic: Educating on Infection Prevention Measures

Education about infection prevention is a crucial role for nurses. One of the most effective ways to prevent the spread of infections, especially in children, is through regular hand hygiene. Therefore, teaching children to wash their hands before meals and after using the bathroom (option 3) is the most appropriate instruction.

Option 1 is incorrect because sharing personal items, especially those that can be contaminated by body fluids such as toothbrushes and towels, can spread infection.

Option 2 is also incorrect as vaccinations are a vital part of preventing the spread of infectious diseases. Avoiding vaccinations can put the child and others at risk of preventable diseases.

Option 4 is incorrect because keeping a sick child at home, even if they're not feeling extremely unwell, can prevent the spread of infection to other students and staff at the school.

For the NCLEX, it's important to understand that teaching effective hand hygiene and promoting vaccinations are key strategies in preventing the spread of infectious diseases. You should also be able to identify incorrect or harmful advice about infection prevention.

Question 41

A nurse is caring for a client who has been demonstrating violent behavior and there is an order to use physical restraints. What is the most appropriate action by the nurse?

1. Apply the restraints and leave the patient alone to calm down.
2. Use the restraints, but check the client's circulation, sensation, and mobility every 15 minutes.
3. Request a security guard to continuously monitor the patient in restraints.
4. Apply the restraints and check on the patient every 2 hours.

Answer Key

The correct answer is 2.

Topic: Use of Restraints

The use of restraints is considered a last-resort intervention to ensure the safety of the client and others, particularly when the client is a risk due to violent or self-harming behavior. Restraints should only be applied under the direction of a healthcare provider and under strict guidelines. Option 2 is the correct answer as it emphasizes the nurse's responsibility in ensuring the client's safety while the restraints are applied. This includes monitoring circulation, sensation, and mobility every 15 minutes.

Option 1 is not appropriate because leaving a patient alone in restraints can lead to serious complications, including injury or death.

Option 3 is incorrect because while a security guard may be necessary in some cases, it is still the nurse's responsibility to assess and monitor the patient's physical and psychological condition.

Option 4 is incorrect because the frequency of checks is insufficient. The patient in restraints needs to be monitored more frequently to prevent potential complications.

Question 42

A nurse is conducting a health promotion teaching session for new parents of a 1-week old infant. Which advice is most appropriate for the nurse to include in the teaching?

1. Start introducing solid foods at around 3 months of age.
2. Put the baby to sleep on his or her back to prevent sudden infant death syndrome.
3. Vaccinations are optional and parents should decide based on personal beliefs.
4. Regular bathing is necessary, at least once a day.

Answer Key

The correct answer is 2.

Topic: Care for Newborns, Infants, and Toddlers

Taking care of newborns, infants, and toddlers is a critical period in a child's development. Nurses play a significant role in educating parents about safe and healthy practices.

Option 2 is the correct answer as it is aligned with the current guidelines by the American Academy of Pediatrics (AAP) regarding sleep positions for infants. The "Back to Sleep" campaign has led to a significant reduction in the occurrence of sudden infant death syndrome (SIDS).

Option 1 is incorrect. The AAP recommends introducing solid foods around 6 months of age, not 3 months.

Option 3 is not accurate. Vaccinations are vital to prevent serious illnesses. Nurses should emphasize the importance of following the recommended vaccination schedule.

Option 4 is not necessary. Newborns and infants do not require daily baths. Over-bathing could lead to skin dryness.

Question 43

A school nurse is educating a group of parents about common health issues in school-aged children. Which of the following should the nurse include as a common health concern in this age group?

1. Respiratory distress due to congenital heart defects.
2. Gastrointestinal disturbances due to dietary changes.
3. Frequent skin infections due to poor personal hygiene.
4. Poor vision and hearing due to genetic factors.

Answer Key
The correct answer is 3.

Topic: Care for Preschool and School Age Clients

Providing care for preschool and school-aged clients often entails a variety of healthcare aspects, including physical health, mental health, growth and development, and health education.

Option 3 is correct. School-aged children are frequently exposed to bacteria and viruses due to their close interaction with peers and their still-developing immune systems. Additionally, children may not always practice good personal hygiene, such as frequent hand washing, which can increase the risk of skin infections.

Option 1 is less likely to be correct as congenital heart defects typically present during infancy or early childhood, and if undiagnosed, could be life-threatening.

Option 2 may not be the most prevalent health issue for school-aged children. Though dietary changes can cause GI disturbances, it is not one of the most common health concerns for this age group.

Option 4 is not the most common health concern for this age group. Though vision and hearing problems can occur due to genetic factors, these issues are not as prevalent as hygiene-related problems.

Question 44

A nurse is caring for a 50-year-old client who reports frequent fatigue and dyspnea on exertion. Which of the following health issues should the nurse consider as the most likely cause?

1. Pneumonia.
2. Type 2 Diabetes Mellitus.
3. Hypertension.
4. Coronary artery disease.

Answer Key
The correct answer is 4.

Topic: Care for Adult Clients (18-64 years)

When it comes to adult clients aged between 18 and 64, nurses need to consider a broad range of potential health issues, including chronic diseases, mental health issues, and age-related changes. The chosen age group typically signifies the period from late adolescence to middle adulthood, a span during which lifestyle-related diseases often begin to manifest.

Option 4, coronary artery disease (CAD), is the correct answer in this scenario. The client's symptoms of fatigue and dyspnea (shortness of breath) on exertion are common signs of CAD. This disease occurs when the major blood vessels that supply the heart with blood, oxygen, and nutrients (coronary arteries) become damaged or diseased.

Option 1, Pneumonia, while can cause fatigue and dyspnea, is usually accompanied by other symptoms such as cough with phlegm, fever, and chills.

Option 2, Type 2 Diabetes Mellitus, can cause fatigue, but dyspnea on exertion is not a typical symptom.

Option 3, Hypertension, usually does not present with symptoms until it's severe and it's often known as a "silent killer".

Question 45

A nurse is working with an 80-year-old client who recently underwent a hip replacement. The client reports difficulty sleeping at night due to discomfort. What is the best nursing intervention in this situation?

1. Offer a warm drink before bedtime.
2. Administer pain medication as ordered.
3. Increase daytime physical activity.
4. Recommend use of a sleep aid.

Answer Key
The correct answer is 2.

Topic: Care for Geriatric Clients (65+ years)

Providing care for geriatric clients (65+ years) requires an understanding of the unique challenges and considerations that come with aging. This often includes managing chronic conditions, decreased physical ability, sensory deficits, and increased susceptibility to acute illnesses and infections.

In this question, the client has undergone a hip replacement and is having difficulty sleeping due to discomfort. This situation is fairly common in geriatric clients following such procedures. Therefore, the most direct and effective intervention would be to administer pain medication as ordered (option 2). It's important to regularly assess the client's pain level and provide pain relief measures to ensure comfort and promote healing.

Option 1, offering a warm drink before bedtime, can sometimes help with sleep, but it is not directly addressing the client's pain.

Option 3, increasing daytime physical activity, may help with sleep but may not be feasible post-surgery and does not directly address the pain.

Option 4, recommending the use of a sleep aid, might not be the best choice given the risk of potential side effects and interactions with other medications the client might be taking.

Preparing for the NCLEX involves understanding that the aging process affects all body systems, which influences how you deliver care and educate elderly clients. Elderly clients may also have different responses to treatments and medications, due to changes in body systems and the presence of multiple chronic conditions. Therefore, a tailored approach is often required when dealing with this population group.

Question 46

A nurse is providing prenatal education to a first-time expectant mother. Which of the following should the nurse include in her teaching?

1. Regular exercise is discouraged during pregnancy.
2. It is normal to have no weight gain during the first trimester.
3. Alcohol should be completely avoided throughout the pregnancy.
4. Frequent consumption of caffeinated beverages is safe during pregnancy.

Answer Key
The correct answer is 3.

Topic: Prenatal Care and Education

Prenatal care and education are essential aspects of nursing practice, especially for expectant mothers who are experiencing pregnancy for the first time. The goal of prenatal care is to provide regular check-ups that allow doctors or midwives to treat and prevent potential health problems throughout the course of the pregnancy while promoting healthy lifestyles that benefit both mother and child.

In this question, the correct answer is 3, which advises the avoidance of alcohol throughout pregnancy. Alcohol consumption during pregnancy can lead to fetal alcohol syndrome and other developmental disorders. This is a universally accepted guideline in prenatal care.

Option 1 is incorrect because moderate-intensity exercise is generally safe and beneficial during pregnancy, unless contraindicated by a healthcare provider.

Option 2 is also incorrect. Although weight gain might vary among individuals, some weight gain (usually around 1 to 4.5 pounds) during the first trimester is typically expected and healthy.

Option 4 is incorrect. While it's not necessary to completely eliminate caffeine, it's recommended that pregnant women limit their caffeine intake due to potential risks.

When preparing for the NCLEX, it's essential to be aware of best practices in prenatal care and education. Understanding the changes that occur during pregnancy and knowing how to guide pregnant women in managing these changes can significantly impact the health outcomes of both the mother and baby.

Question 47

A nurse is monitoring a client who is in labor. Which of the following changes should alert the nurse to possible labor complications?

1. Contractions lasting 45-60 seconds and occurring every 3-5 minutes.
2. An increase in bloody show.
3. A sudden decrease in the intensity of contractions.
4. An increase in the client's level of discomfort.

Answer Key
The correct answer is 3.

Topic: Antepartum and Labor Client Care

Antepartum and labor care encompasses nursing interventions during the antepartum period (before childbirth) and labor (the process of childbirth). It's crucial to closely monitor both the mother and fetus during this period to ensure a safe and healthy delivery.

In this question, the correct answer is 3: A sudden decrease in the intensity of contractions could signify a problem such as uterine rupture or placental abruption. Both conditions are serious and require immediate medical attention.

Option 1 is incorrect as contractions that last 45-60 seconds and occur every 3-5 minutes are normal during active labor.

Option 2 is also incorrect. An increase in bloody show, or the discharge of mucus and blood from the vagina, is a normal sign of progressing labor.

Option 4 is incorrect as an increase in discomfort level is to be expected during labor. However, extreme pain or sudden changes in pain should be evaluated.

As you prepare for the NCLEX, understanding the stages of labor and being able to identify potential complications is vital. Nurses play an instrumental role in the labor and delivery process and must have the knowledge and skills to identify and respond to any deviations from the normal labor process.

Question 48

A nurse is providing postpartum care to a client who has just given birth. Which of the following findings should the nurse report immediately?

1. The client has a temperature of 37.2 C (99 F).
2. The client expresses feelings of joy and relief.
3. The client's uterus is firm, midline and at the level of the umbilicus.
4. The client's perineal pad is saturated within one hour after birth.

Answer Key
The correct answer is 4.

Topic: Post-Partum Care and Education

Postpartum care refers to the care provided to the mother following childbirth. This period is a time of physiological and psychological readjustment for the woman, and also a time when the new mother needs to learn the skills necessary to care for her newborn.

In the given question, the correct answer is 4. A perineal pad becoming saturated within an hour after birth is a concerning sign of postpartum hemorrhage, a potentially life-threatening complication that requires immediate medical intervention.

Option 1 is incorrect because a temperature of 37.2 C (99 F) is within the normal range.

Option 2 is also incorrect because feelings of joy and relief are normal emotions for a new mother to experience following childbirth.

Option 3 is incorrect because a firm, midline uterus at the level of the umbilicus is an expected finding in the immediate postpartum period.

As you prepare for the NCLEX, remember that recognizing postpartum complications like hemorrhage is a critical aspect of nursing care. The nurse's role in postpartum care includes monitoring the mother's physical condition, providing education on infant care and self-care, supporting breastfeeding, and assessing the mother's emotional well-being.

Question 49

A public health nurse is conducting a community health risk assessment. Which of the following data should be collected for this assessment?

1. Individual health histories of all community members.
2. The number of fast-food restaurants in the area.
3. The voting patterns of the community in the last election.
4. The average salary of individuals in the community.

Answer Key
The correct answer is 2.

Topic: Health Risk Assessments Based on Family, Community

In public health, a community health risk assessment is a systematic approach to identifying and analyzing the health risks of a specific community. This process involves collecting data related to various determinants of health, including environmental, biological, and lifestyle factors.

Option 2 is the correct answer because the number of fast-food restaurants in an area can have significant implications for the dietary habits and consequently, the overall health of the community. A high density of fast-food restaurants may be associated with higher rates of obesity, cardiovascular disease, and other diet-related health conditions.

Option 1 is incorrect because, while individual health histories can be informative, it's not feasible or necessarily ethical to collect this type of data from all community members for a community-wide health assessment.

Option 3 is incorrect because voting patterns, while potentially indicative of social and political factors within a community, don't directly relate to community health risks.

Option 4 is incorrect because while socioeconomic status can influence health, the average salary of individuals does not directly represent a health risk.

Question 50

A nurse is preparing an educational session for a client recently diagnosed with diabetes. Which of the following is the MOST important assessment the nurse should perform prior to developing the teaching plan?

1. The client's favorite hobbies.
2. The client's preferred learning style.
3. The client's shoe size.
4. The number of friends the client has.

Answer Key
The correct answer is 2.

Topic: Learning Readiness, Preferences, and Barriers Assessment

When educating a client, it's crucial to assess their learning readiness, preferences, and any barriers to learning. This enables the nurse to tailor the teaching plan to best meet the client's needs and optimize their understanding and adherence.

Option 2 is correct because understanding a client's preferred learning style (auditory, visual, kinesthetic, etc.) allows the nurse to present information in the way that the client learns best. This increases the likelihood of the client retaining the information and successfully managing their health condition.

Option 1, while it may provide useful information about the client's personal life, does not directly contribute to developing an effective teaching plan.

Option 3 is irrelevant to developing a teaching plan unless the education is specifically about foot care, which is not indicated in the question.

Option 4 is not directly related to the client's learning readiness or preferences and would not significantly impact the development of a teaching plan.

Question 51

A community health nurse is planning a health education program for a local community. Which of the following actions should the nurse take FIRST?

1. Set the date and time for the program.
2. Evaluate the effectiveness of the program.
3. Determine the health needs and concerns of the community.
4. Design the educational materials for the program.

Answer Key
The correct answer is 3.

Topic: Community Health Education

Community health education is a critical component of public health nursing. Its purpose is to promote, maintain, and improve individual and community health by assisting individuals and communities to adopt healthy behaviors.

Option 3 is correct because, before planning a health education program, the nurse should first determine the health needs and concerns of the community. This ensures that the program addresses the most relevant and significant health issues faced by the community, making it more likely to be effective and well-received.

Option 1 is not the first step in planning a health education program. While scheduling is important, it should occur after determining the community's needs and the program's content.

Option 2, evaluating the effectiveness of the program, is an important step but should be performed after the program has been implemented, not before.

Option 4, designing the educational materials, should occur after identifying the community's health needs to ensure the materials are relevant and targeted.

For the NCLEX exam, it's important to remember the steps involved in planning a community health education program. Understanding the community's health needs is the first step, followed by designing a program to address those needs, implementing the program, and finally, evaluating the effectiveness of the program.

Question 52

A nurse is providing education to a client about the importance of preventative health care. Which of the following points should the nurse stress the MOST?

1. Preventative care can only be achieved through annual check-ups.
2. Preventative care involves eating a balanced diet and regular exercise.
3. Preventative care is unnecessary if the client feels healthy.
4. Preventative care primarily involves using medications to prevent future illnesses.

Answer Key
The correct answer is 2.

Topic: Preventative Care and Health Maintenance

Preventative care and health maintenance are crucial aspects of healthcare. They focus on maintaining health and preventing the onset of diseases rather than treating them after they have developed.

Option 2 is the correct answer because preventative care indeed involves adopting healthy lifestyle habits, such as eating a balanced diet and engaging in regular physical activity. These actions can help prevent many chronic diseases like diabetes, heart disease, and some types of cancer.

Option 1 is incorrect because preventative care is more than just annual check-ups. While regular health check-ups play a vital role in early detection of potential health issues, preventative care is a broader concept that also includes healthy lifestyle habits.

Option 3 is not correct as preventative care is necessary even when a person feels healthy. Many diseases can develop and progress without causing noticeable symptoms until they reach advanced stages.

Option 4 is incorrect because while some preventative measures might include medications (like vaccines or preventive drugs for conditions like malaria), it's not the primary focus. The main goal of preventative care is to promote overall health and prevent disease through healthy habits and regular screenings.

For the NCLEX exam, it's essential to understand that preventative care and health maintenance encompass a wide range of health behaviors, including diet, exercise, and regular health screenings. All of these factors contribute to preventing the onset of disease and maintaining optimal health.

Question 53

A nurse is communicating with a client who speaks very little English. Which of the following strategies should the nurse use to MINIMIZE communication barriers?

1. Speak louder and slower.
2. Use a certified interpreter.
3. Use medical jargon to explain the condition.
4. Ask the client's family member to translate.

Answer Key
The correct answer is 2.

Topic: Communication Barrier Minimization

Minimizing communication barriers is crucial for effective nursing care. When the client and healthcare provider do not share a common language, this can present significant challenges in conveying and understanding medical information.

Option 2 is the correct answer because using a certified interpreter ensures accurate translation and preserves the confidentiality of the client's health information.

Option 1 is incorrect as speaking louder and slower may not aid in comprehension if the client does not understand the language. Moreover, it can come across as disrespectful or condescending.

Option 3 is not correct because using medical jargon can exacerbate the communication barrier, even when speaking with clients who share the same language as the healthcare provider. It's always essential to use layman's terms that the client can understand.

Option 4 is incorrect because family members might not accurately translate medical information due to a lack of medical knowledge. In addition, using family members as translators can breach the client's confidentiality.

For the NCLEX exam, understanding the importance of effective communication, respecting cultural diversity, and upholding the client's rights to privacy and confidentiality are vital. Always consider using professional interpreters when language barriers exist, and ensure information is conveyed in a manner the client can understand.

Question 54

A nurse is working in a community health center. Which of the following clients should be prioritized for a targeted screening assessment?

1. A 50-year-old male with no family history of disease and no complaints.
2. A 35-year-old female with a family history of breast cancer.
3. A 21-year-old male athlete with a history of multiple strains.
4. A 68-year-old female who has had a complete physical examination last year.

Answer Key
The correct answer is 2.

Topic: Targeted Screening Assessments

Targeted screening assessments refer to a methodical approach to detect diseases or conditions in individuals who appear to be at high risk. This approach is often utilized in individuals who have certain risk factors but are asymptomatic.

Option 2 is the correct answer as the client has a family history of breast cancer, which significantly increases her risk. Therefore, she should be prioritized for a targeted screening assessment like mammography.

Option 1, the 50-year-old male with no family history of disease or complaints, may not necessarily need a targeted screening unless there were specific risk factors present.

Option 3, the 21-year-old male athlete, without any significant complaints, also would not necessarily need a targeted screening.

Option 4, the 68-year-old female who had a complete physical examination last year, would only need targeted screenings if there were changes in her risk profile since her last check-up or if she was not up to date with screenings.

Question 55

A nurse is providing care for a patient who has a history of heavy smoking and alcohol consumption. Which of the following strategies is most appropriate for the nurse to use in addressing these high-risk health behaviors?

1. Encourage the patient to immediately quit smoking and drinking.
2. Assist the patient in setting realistic goals for reducing smoking and alcohol consumption.
3. Ignore the behaviors unless the patient brings them up.
4. Encourage the patient to replace smoking and drinking with another habit.

Answer Key
The correct answer is 2.

Topic: High Risk Health Behavior Prevention and Treatment

High risk health behaviors such as excessive smoking and alcohol consumption can lead to serious health consequences. Nurses play a crucial role in preventing and treating these behaviors through patient education, counseling, and by providing resources for behavioral changes.

Option 2 is the best approach as it assists the patient in setting realistic and achievable goals to reduce harmful behaviors. Immediate cessation of smoking and alcohol (Option 1) can be unrealistic and potentially dangerous due to withdrawal symptoms. Ignoring the behaviors (Option 3) is not ethical or helpful as nurses have an obligation to address harmful behaviors with their patients. Replacing smoking and drinking with another habit (Option 4) can potentially lead to new harmful habits.

When studying for the NCLEX exam, remember that nurses should promote a harm reduction approach that helps patients move towards healthier habits at their own pace. Patient education and collaboration are key in supporting behavior change.

Question 56

A nurse is caring for a patient who recently underwent a hip replacement surgery and is now transitioning to home care. What is the most important consideration for the nurse when managing the patient's care in the home environment?

1. Making sure the home is a comfortable place for the patient.
2. Ensuring there is a caregiver at home to support the patient.
3. Assessing and adapting the home environment for safety and accessibility.
4. Confirming the patient's home address and contact information.

Answer Key
The correct answer is 3.

Topic: Managing Care in Home Environment

When transitioning to home care after a hospital stay, especially after surgeries like a hip replacement, it is vital to ensure that the home environment is adapted for safety and accessibility to prevent falls and promote independence.

Option 1 is important but not the primary concern, as the comfort of a home does not necessarily ensure its safety or accessibility. Having a caregiver at home (Option 2) can be extremely beneficial, but it does not replace the necessity of a safe and accessible environment. Confirming the patient's home address and contact information (Option 4) is part of administrative work and does not directly impact the management of care in the home environment.

While preparing for the NCLEX exam, remember that a significant part of home care nursing is the initial home visit where the nurse assesses the environment, identifies potential risks, and makes necessary recommendations for modifications. The goal is to create a safe, functional environment that supports the patient's recovery and well-being.

Question 57

A nurse is conducting a comprehensive health assessment for a new patient. Which of the following actions is most appropriate for the nurse to take?

1. Focusing primarily on the patient's presenting symptoms.
2. Gathering information only about the patient's medical history.
3. Including an assessment of the patient's mental and social health.
4. Documenting only the physical examination findings.

Answer Key
The correct answer is 3.

Topic: Comprehensive Health Assessments

Comprehensive health assessments are a crucial part of nursing care. They are foundational in establishing a thorough understanding of the patient's health status, which informs the planning and implementation of individualized care. The scope of these assessments is broad and encompasses various aspects of the patient's health, including physical, psychological, sociocultural, and spiritual dimensions.

In the NCLEX exam, it's crucial to recognize that comprehensive health assessments involve more than just a focus on the patient's presenting symptoms (Option 1) or a documentation of the physical examination findings (Option 4). These are important elements, but they form only part of the picture. A truly comprehensive assessment looks beyond these elements, exploring the patient's overall well-being and identifying potential health risks.

Option 2, gathering information only about the patient's medical history, is also not considered comprehensive. While a patient's medical history is an essential aspect of the assessment, it should not be the sole focus. An effective comprehensive health assessment requires a broader view that includes current lifestyle factors, family history, and environmental factors that may affect the patient's health.

Answer 3 best embodies the concept of a comprehensive health assessment. Mental and social health are integral to a patient's overall well-being and should always be included in the assessment. Mental health conditions can affect a patient's ability to cope with physical illnesses, while social health aspects, such as support systems and living conditions, can influence health outcomes. By considering these factors, nurses can develop a more holistic and effective plan of care.

As you prepare for the NCLEX exam, it's crucial to understand the importance of comprehensive health assessments. Remember, the main goal of these assessments is to gather complete and detailed information about the patient, which serves as a basis for planning and delivering individualized, patient-centered care. Understanding the patient as a whole - their physical health, mental and emotional state, social environment, and even spiritual beliefs - allows the nurse to provide care that is truly aligned with the patient's needs and preferences. This not only improves the quality of care but also enhances patient satisfaction and health outcomes.

Question 58

A nurse is caring for a child in the pediatric unit. Which of the following observations should most alert the nurse to a possible case of neglect?

1. The child is overly friendly and open to all hospital staff.
2. The child has poor hygiene and is underweight.
3. The child is often seen playing with other children in the ward.
4. The child's parents always bring in the child's favorite meals.

Answer Key
The correct answer is 2.

Topic: Assessing for Abuse or Neglect

Abuse or neglect assessment is a highly sensitive and important area in nursing. In such assessments, the nurse must be aware of the signs that may indicate a child, adult, or elderly person is experiencing abuse or neglect. Understanding these indicators can lead to early detection and interventions, potentially saving a person from further harm.

Neglect, a form of child maltreatment, is defined as the failure by the caregiver to provide needed, age-appropriate care despite the financial ability to do so. Signs of neglect can vary and may include observations of poor hygiene, inadequate nutrition, lack of supervision, or failure to provide necessary medical treatment.

In this context, option 2, observing that the child has poor hygiene and is underweight, can be a clear sign of neglect. These could suggest that the child is not receiving adequate care, including proper nutrition and personal hygiene, from their caregiver.

The other options may not necessarily suggest neglect. A child being overly friendly (option 1) can be a characteristic of their personality. Seeing a child play with other children (option 3) is generally a good sign of social development. The fact that parents bring their child's favorite meals (option 4) indicates their concern for the child's well-being and specific preferences.

On the NCLEX exam, it's important to recall these indicators and interpret them within the given context. Remember, if you suspect a child or any patient is a victim of abuse or neglect, it's crucial to report it to the proper authorities as required by your state's laws. In many cases, nurses are mandated reporters, meaning they have a legal obligation to report suspected abuse or neglect. These actions align with the fundamental ethical responsibility of nurses to advocate for their patient's safety and welfare. Keep this in mind as you prepare for your NCLEX exam and your future nursing practice.

Question 59

A nurse is caring for a client who has been diagnosed with bipolar disorder and is exhibiting manic behavior. Which of the following behavioral management techniques should the nurse utilize?

1. Encourage the client to participate in numerous group activities to help distract them.
2. Maintain a calm, quiet environment and limit stimuli.
3. Allow the client to make decisions regarding their care to help them regain control.
4. Provide detailed explanations of procedures to help ease the client's anxiety.

Answer Key
The correct answer is 2.

Topic: Behavioral Management Techniques in Care

Behavioral management techniques are essential tools for nurses in dealing with clients exhibiting various forms of behaviors, including those related to mental health disorders such as bipolar disorder.

In bipolar disorder, clients may go through manic phases where they exhibit hyperactivity, rapid speech, and may easily be distracted. During these times, the priority is to provide a stable, calm, and quiet environment that helps them stay grounded and prevent overstimulation, which is why option 2 is the correct answer.

Option 1 is incorrect because encouraging the client to participate in numerous group activities may overwhelm them and exacerbate their manic symptoms.

Option 3 is not the best choice. While it's essential to involve clients in care decisions, during a manic phase, a client might struggle with decision-making due to heightened impulsivity.

Option 4, providing detailed explanations, may not be effective because clients in a manic phase often struggle with attention and may not fully grasp complex information.

Understanding behavioral management techniques for different mental health disorders is crucial for the NCLEX exam and your future nursing practice. This involves recognizing the specific needs and behaviors of clients with different conditions and knowing the appropriate interventions to provide a supportive, therapeutic environment for them.

In your studies, remember that each patient is unique, and their care should be individualized. The techniques you use should always be in the best interest of promoting safety and improving the client's overall well-being. Also, these techniques should be evidence-based, as the field of mental health is continuously evolving with new research.

Using these techniques effectively not only contributes to positive patient outcomes but also helps to build a strong therapeutic nurse-patient relationship, which is an essential component of comprehensive nursing care.

Question 60

A nurse is conducting an assessment on a client who has a history of substance abuse. The client has not been forthcoming about their substance use. Which of the following strategies should the nurse use to facilitate a more open conversation about substance abuse?

1. Confront the client about inconsistencies in their statements.
2. Ask open-ended questions to encourage the client to share their experiences.
3. Threaten to inform law enforcement if the client does not confess.
4. Tell the client about the health risks associated with substance abuse.

Answer Key
The correct answer is 2.

Topic: Substance Abuse Assessment and Intervention

Substance abuse assessment and intervention is a critical component of nursing care. In this case, the nurse needs to build a non-judgmental and therapeutic rapport with the client to facilitate an open and honest discussion about the client's substance abuse.

The correct answer is option 2: asking open-ended questions. This strategy encourages the client to share more about their experiences, feelings, and concerns, making the conversation more client-centered and therapeutic.

Option 1, confronting the client, might provoke defensiveness and hinder the establishment of a therapeutic rapport.

Option 3, threatening to inform law enforcement, violates the client's rights and breaks trust. Confidentiality is a key ethical principle in nursing, and threats undermine the therapeutic relationship.

Option 4, while educating the client on the health risks associated with substance abuse is important, it is more critical to first establish a safe and trustful environment to facilitate this conversation.

When studying for the NCLEX, it's essential to understand that these sensitive discussions must be held in a non-threatening, empathetic, and supportive environment. This allows the client to feel safe enough to disclose their substance use and work collaboratively with the nurse to plan for interventions.

Nurses also need to be aware of their own attitudes and biases towards substance use and ensure these do not negatively impact their approach to care. Knowledge of community resources and referral systems is also crucial, as these clients often require further support and treatment beyond the initial intervention.

Effective substance abuse assessment and intervention involve comprehensive patient education, individualized care planning, ongoing evaluation and adjustment of the care plan, and collaboration with a multidisciplinary team, including addiction specialists, social workers, and mental health professionals.

This approach not only addresses the immediate medical needs of the client but also contributes to their long-term recovery and health. Remember, recovery is a journey, not a destination, and each client's journey will be unique. Your role as a nurse is to support this journey, promoting health and well-being at every stage.

Question 61

A nurse is providing care to a client who recently experienced the loss of a spouse. The client is showing signs of difficulty coping with this major life change. Which of the following interventions should the nurse implement first?

1. Encourage the client to seek psychiatric treatment.
2. Instruct the client to participate in group therapy.
3. Listen empathetically to the client's feelings about the loss.
4. Provide the client with reading materials about grief and loss.

Answer Key
The correct answer is 3.

Topic: Coping with Life Changes

Helping clients cope with major life changes is a common and crucial aspect of nursing care. It's important to understand that the process of coping with life changes is unique for every individual and depends on various factors such as personality traits, personal values, social support, and previous experiences.

The correct answer is option 3: listening empathetically to the client's feelings about the loss. When dealing with individuals undergoing significant life changes, the first step should always be to provide emotional support and validation. By listening empathetically, the nurse establishes a trusting relationship, validates the client's emotions, and encourages the client to express their feelings.

Option 1, encouraging the client to seek psychiatric treatment, and option 2, instructing the client to participate in group therapy, may eventually be part of the client's care plan. However, before suggesting these interventions, it's crucial to first assess the client's current emotional state and coping abilities.

Option 4, providing the client with reading materials about grief and loss, can also be a beneficial strategy. However, it's important to first allow the client to express their emotions and then offer this information as a resource.

For the NCLEX, remember that therapeutic communication is at the heart of nursing. By providing empathetic listening, you create a safe and comforting environment that enables the client to cope better with their situation. It's also crucial to note that while nurses play an important role in providing emotional support, collaboration with mental health professionals may also be necessary in complex cases or if the client exhibits signs of prolonged or complicated grief.

Lastly, the nurse's role also includes educating clients and their families about healthy coping strategies, community resources, and when professional help might be necessary. This holistic approach to care ensures that clients receive the support they need to navigate life changes successfully.

Question 62

A nurse is working in an emergency department and assessing a client who is acting increasingly agitated and aggressive. Which of the following actions should the nurse take FIRST to assess the client's potential for violence?

1. Call security to restrain the client.
2. Obtain a detailed psychiatric history.
3. Implement therapeutic communication techniques.
4. Determine if the client has any personal belongings that could be used as weapons.

Answer Key
The correct answer is 3.

Topic: Violence Potential Assessment and Safety Precautions

Assessing the potential for violence in clients is a critical component of providing safe, quality care. In situations where a client demonstrates escalating agitation and aggressive behaviors, nurses must rapidly evaluate the potential for violence and implement appropriate safety precautions.

The correct answer is option 3: implementing therapeutic communication techniques. Engaging the client in a calm, respectful, and non-confrontational manner can deescalate the situation, build trust, and provide an opportunity to gather information about the client's current emotional state and thoughts.

Option 1, calling security to restrain the client, should be a last resort after all other de-escalation techniques have been exhausted. Restraints can escalate aggression, infringe on client rights, and should only be used when the client is a direct threat to self or others, and less restrictive interventions have been ineffective.

Option 2, obtaining a detailed psychiatric history, is important but may not be feasible immediately in an emergent situation. The nurse's initial focus should be on stabilizing the immediate situation.

Option 4, determining if the client has any personal belongings that could be used as weapons, is a crucial safety precaution but should be pursued in a careful, non-provocative manner, ideally after initial engagement and de-escalation attempts.

Remember that on the NCLEX and in practice, client and staff safety is paramount. Therefore, understanding how to assess for potential violence and employing strategies to deescalate volatile situations are key skills. Additionally, early identification of potential risks, close monitoring of clients showing signs of agitation, maintaining clear communication with the healthcare team, and establishing a safe environment are critical elements of care. Moreover, always be aware of your facility's policies and protocols for handling potentially violent situations.

Question 63

A nurse is providing care to a recently admitted patient of Hmong origin who appears distressed. The patient's family requests the presence of a "Txiv Neeb" (Hmong shaman) to perform a traditional healing ceremony. How should the nurse respond?

1. Deny the request because it goes against hospital policy.
2. Allow the request because it is essential to respect the cultural practices of the patient.
3. Ask the family to explain the significance of the ceremony.
4. Inform the family that the ceremony can be performed only after discharge.

Answer Key
The correct answer is 2.

Topic: Incorporating Cultural Practices in Care

Understanding and respecting a client's cultural beliefs and practices are essential aspects of providing comprehensive, person-centered care.

The correct answer is option 2: allowing the request because it is essential to respect the cultural practices of the patient. Nurses are expected to advocate for their patients and facilitate care that is respectful of and responsive to the cultural and religious beliefs and practices that support health and well-being.

Option 1, denying the request because it goes against hospital policy, may not be the right choice without first exploring the possibilities of accommodation. Hospitals should have policies to accommodate cultural and religious practices as long as they do not pose a risk to patient health.

Option 3, asking the family to explain the significance of the ceremony, while valuable for expanding the nurse's understanding and establishing rapport, does not directly address the request. The immediate need is to respond to the family's request, and further inquiry can follow.

Option 4, informing the family that the ceremony can only be performed after discharge, may unnecessarily delay a practice that could potentially contribute to the patient's sense of well-being and recovery.

When preparing for the NCLEX, remember that culturally competent care, including incorporating cultural practices in care, is an important topic. Culturally competent care enhances communication, fosters a mutual respect between the nurse and client, and results in improved patient outcomes. A nurse's ability to recognize, respect, and accommodate patients' cultural practices is an integral aspect of person-centered care.

Question 64

A hospice nurse is caring for a patient with advanced lung cancer. The patient is experiencing severe dyspnea and expresses fear about the dying process. What should be the nurse's initial response?

1. Assure the patient that modern pain management can keep them comfortable.
2. Encourage the patient to talk about their fears and feelings.
3. Explain the biological process of dying to reassure the patient.
4. Recommend the patient to speak with a spiritual counselor.

Answer Key
The correct answer is 2.

Topic: End-of-Life Care and Education

End-of-life care is a crucial topic on the NCLEX and a significant aspect of nursing. This care focuses on providing support, comfort, and relief from pain and other distressing symptoms to patients who are in the advanced stages of a disease leading to death.

The correct answer, in this case, is option 2: encouraging the patient to talk about their fears and feelings. This response demonstrates the nurse's role in providing emotional support and validating the patient's feelings. Engaging in such conversations can help alleviate anxiety and provide a sense of relief to the patient.

Option 1, assuring the patient that modern pain management can keep them comfortable, although partly correct, is not the best initial response as it does not address the patient's expressed fear about dying.

Option 3, explaining the biological process of dying to reassure the patient, can be useful in some cases, but this should be done cautiously, taking into account the patient's readiness and willingness to discuss such details.

Option 4, recommending the patient to speak with a spiritual counselor, is a good choice if the patient expresses a need for spiritual support. Still, it should not replace the nurse's role in offering emotional support.

When studying for the NCLEX, remember that the patient's psychosocial needs, including the need to discuss their feelings and fears, are as important as their physical needs in end-of-life care. Effective communication is a significant part of this process, along with pain management, symptom control, psychological, and spiritual care.

Question 65

A nurse is providing care for a client who recently lost his job and is showing signs of depression. The nurse is assessing the client's support system. Which of the following actions should the nurse take FIRST?

1. Arrange a consultation with a psychiatrist for medication management.
2. Recommend the client attend a support group for individuals with depression.
3. Ask the client about their current social connections and relationships.
4. Discuss the option of psychotherapy with the client.

Answer Key

The correct answer is 3.

Topic: Assessing Client Support System

Assessing a client's support system is an integral part of nursing care and a significant topic on the NCLEX exam. A strong support system can play a vital role in a client's physical and mental well-being, particularly during times of stress or illness.

The correct answer is option 3: asking the client about their current social connections and relationships. This action allows the nurse to gain insight into the client's support system, which could include friends, family, or close associates. Understanding the client's support system is essential in determining how they may cope with their current situation and any potential stressors.

Option 1, arranging a consultation with a psychiatrist for medication management, is a potential intervention, but the nurse first needs to understand the client's support system to inform any interventions.

Option 2, recommending the client attend a support group for individuals with depression, is a useful intervention for some clients but again should follow a comprehensive assessment of the client's social support system.

Option 4, discussing the option of psychotherapy with the client, is also an intervention that might be appropriate but should be guided by a thorough understanding of the client's support system and personal preferences.

In preparation for the NCLEX, remember the importance of assessing the client's support system before planning and implementing interventions. These assessments can guide interventions and provide valuable insights into the client's capacity for coping with adversity. Always consider the "Assessment" before "Implementation" when answering NCLEX questions.

Question 66

A nurse is caring for a client who just lost a loved one. Which of the following statements by the nurse would be MOST appropriate in providing care for this grieving client?

1. "I know exactly how you're feeling. I lost someone very close to me last year."
2. "Why don't you try and distract yourself with some activities to take your mind off your grief?"
3. "Your loved one is in a better place now."
4. "I'm here to support you. It's okay to express your feelings and emotions."

Answer Key
The correct answer is 4.

Topic: Providing Care for Grieving Clients

Providing care for grieving clients is a sensitive and crucial topic on the NCLEX exam and an integral part of nursing practice. Nurses must know how to communicate empathetically and provide the necessary emotional support. The correct answer is option 4: "I'm here to support you. It's okay to express your feelings and emotions." This statement shows empathy, respect, and a willingness to support the client during their grieving process. It validates the client's feelings and reassures them that expressing their emotions is natural and healthy during this difficult time.

Option 1, "I know exactly how you're feeling. I lost someone very close to me last year," may seem empathetic, but it's generally not helpful to assume that you know exactly how another person is feeling. Each person's experience with grief is unique, and this statement could unintentionally minimize the client's feelings.

Option 2, "Why don't you try and distract yourself with some activities to take your mind off your grief?" may be inappropriate as it might be perceived as ignoring or invalidating the client's feelings of grief.

Option 3, "Your loved one is in a better place now." may conflict with the client's personal beliefs or feelings about the situation, potentially causing additional distress.

As you prepare for the NCLEX exam, it's important to remember that empathy and understanding are fundamental to caring for grieving clients. Always validate and respect the client's feelings and emotions, and offer support in a nonjudgmental and caring manner. Understanding and applying these principles will be key in answering questions on this topic successfully.

Question 67

A nurse is providing care to a client who was recently diagnosed with bipolar disorder, a chronic psychosocial health issue. Which of the following interventions should the nurse consider as a priority in this client's care plan?

1. Encouraging the client to engage in regular physical activity to manage symptoms.
2. Encouraging the client to stop taking prescribed medication when symptoms subside.
3. Educating the client about the importance of regular follow-up with the mental health team.
4. Encouraging the client to avoid discussing their diagnosis with friends and family to avoid stigmatization.

Answer Key
The correct answer is 3.

Topic: Acute and Chronic Psychosocial Health Issues

Acute and chronic psychosocial health issues constitute a significant portion of the NCLEX exam and are crucial in real-world nursing practice. Nurses play an essential role in educating clients, providing supportive care, and advocating for clients' rights.

The correct answer is option 3, "Educating the client about the importance of regular follow-up with the mental health team." Regular follow-up and communication with mental health professionals are vital in managing chronic psychosocial disorders like bipolar disorder. These healthcare providers are equipped to assess the effectiveness of treatment plans, adjust medication regimens as necessary, provide therapeutic interventions, and support clients in managing their condition.

Option 1, "Encouraging the client to engage in regular physical activity to manage symptoms," is beneficial as part of a holistic approach to managing bipolar disorder, but it's not the priority. Physical activity alone cannot manage the symptoms of bipolar disorder.

Option 2, "Encouraging the client to stop taking prescribed medication when symptoms subside," is incorrect. It is

195

essential to adhere to medication regimens, even when symptoms appear to improve. Abruptly stopping medication can lead to a relapse or exacerbation of symptoms.

Option 4, "Encouraging the client to avoid discussing their diagnosis with friends and family to avoid stigmatization," is not recommended. Clients should be encouraged to communicate openly about their condition to foster a support system.

In the context of the NCLEX and nursing practice, understanding the importance of regular follow-ups, medication adherence, supportive communication, and a holistic approach to care are vital for clients with psychosocial health issues. This knowledge will not only help in answering NCLEX questions correctly but also in providing quality care to clients.

Question 68

A nurse is providing care to a client who recently immigrated to the United States. The client's cultural beliefs and traditions differ significantly from the nurse's. Which of the following actions is the most appropriate way for the nurse to provide care?

1. The nurse should disregard the client's cultural beliefs and provide care based on her understanding.
2. The nurse should insist on strictly adhering to the client's cultural practices even if they conflict with medical recommendations.
3. The nurse should seek to understand and incorporate the client's cultural beliefs into the care plan, in consultation with the healthcare team.
4. The nurse should rely solely on the client's family for all decisions related to care due to the cultural differences.

Answer Key
The correct answer is 3.

Topic: Psychosocial Factors Influencing Care

Psychosocial factors significantly impact the way care is provided and received. Recognizing these factors is crucial to offer individualized, culturally appropriate, and effective care. This topic is an essential aspect of the NCLEX exam and everyday nursing practice.

The correct answer is option 3, "The nurse should seek to understand and incorporate the client's cultural beliefs into the care plan, in consultation with the healthcare team." This approach respects the client's autonomy and cultural beliefs while ensuring the medical needs are met. It's about balancing cultural competence and medical necessity.

Option 1, "The nurse should disregard the client's cultural beliefs and provide care based on her understanding," is not recommended. This approach is ethnocentric and does not respect the client's cultural beliefs and individuality.

Option 2, "The nurse should insist on strictly adhering to the client's cultural practices even if they conflict with medical recommendations," is also not suitable. While it's important to respect a client's cultural beliefs, healthcare professionals must ensure the client's safety and wellbeing. They should negotiate with the client to find a middle ground that respects their cultural practices and ensures their health needs are met.

Option 4, "The nurse should rely solely on the client's family for all decisions related to care due to the cultural differences," is not recommended. While family members can play an important role in decision-making, the client's autonomy and rights to participate in their care should not be overlooked.

For the NCLEX and in nursing practice, understanding how to navigate cultural differences and incorporate these considerations into care planning is critical. It promotes respectful, person-centered care, which leads to better health outcomes and client satisfaction.

Question 69

A nurse is caring for a client with advanced Alzheimer's disease. The client is having difficulty remembering family members and is becoming increasingly agitated. Which of the following is the most appropriate intervention for the nurse to implement?

1. Isolate the client to prevent him from becoming more agitated.
2. Constantly remind the client about the family members he can't remember.
3. Use validation therapy, reassuring the client and exploring his feelings and thoughts.
4. Insist that the client must try harder to remember things.

Answer Key
The correct answer is 3.

Topic: Caring for Clients with Sensory or Cognitive Alterations

Caring for clients with sensory or cognitive alterations, such as Alzheimer's disease, requires special consideration, empathy, and a unique set of nursing interventions. This area is important for the NCLEX as it demands a broad understanding of neurocognitive disorders and effective care strategies.

The correct answer is option 3: "Use validation therapy, reassuring the client and exploring his feelings and thoughts." Validation therapy is an empathetic way of managing clients with cognitive impairments. The therapy does not argue with or correct the patient's perceptions; instead, it validates their experiences and emotions, promoting communication and reducing agitation.

Option 1, "Isolate the client to prevent him from becoming more agitated," is not recommended. Isolation can cause further agitation, loneliness, and confusion.

Option 2, "Constantly remind the client about the family members he can't remember," is not helpful either. This can lead to frustration, anxiety, and increased agitation for the client. It's better to introduce family members gently, provide reassurance, and create a calm and supportive environment. Option 4, "Insist that the client must try harder to remember things," is incorrect. This approach may increase the client's frustration and anxiety levels. It's not about the client not trying hard enough; Alzheimer's disease is a progressive condition that affects memory.

To prepare for NCLEX and provide effective nursing care, understanding the unique needs of clients with sensory or cognitive alterations is essential. Therapies like validation and reminiscence, creating a safe and familiar environment, and maintaining a calm demeanor can greatly improve the quality of care for these clients.

Question 70

A nurse is caring for a patient who recently lost his job due to chronic illness. Despite the patient maintaining a positive verbal demeanor, the nurse notices signs of distress. Which of the following non-verbal cues should the nurse identify as an indication of stress?

1. The patient maintains consistent eye contact during the conversation.
2. The patient frequently sighs and has a slumped posture.
3. The patient keeps a regular sleeping schedule.
4. The patient's heart rate and blood pressure are within normal range.

Answer Key
The correct answer is 2.

Topic: Recognizing Non-Verbal Cues to Stressors

Recognizing non-verbal cues to stressors is a vital skill for nurses, and it's a topic covered in the NCLEX exam. This ability helps nurses identify when a patient may be experiencing emotional distress, even if they're not openly expressing it.

In this question, the correct answer is option 2: "The patient frequently sighs and has a slumped posture." These are classic non-verbal signs of stress. Sighing often indicates feelings of sadness or frustration, while a slumped posture can signal low energy or feelings of defeat.

Option 1, maintaining consistent eye contact, does not typically indicate stress. Rather, it's often seen as a sign of engagement in the conversation.

Option 3, keeping a regular sleeping schedule, is a positive sign and typically indicative of good health and well-being.

Option 4, having normal heart rate and blood pressure, does not necessarily correlate with a person's stress level, as these can be within normal range even in stressful conditions, depending on the individual's coping mechanisms.

As a nurse preparing for the NCLEX, recognizing non-verbal cues can aid in holistic care delivery. By paying attention to these subtle signs, nurses can initiate conversations about stress, provide emotional support, and intervene as necessary. It's all part of providing comprehensive care and addressing not only a patient's physical needs but also their mental and emotional well-being.

Question 71

A nurse is caring for a patient who is anxious about an upcoming surgery. Which of the following therapeutic communication techniques is most appropriate for the nurse to use in this situation?

1. Giving advice about what the patient should do to feel less anxious.
2. Telling the patient that everything will be okay and there is no need to worry.
3. Encouraging the patient to talk about his feelings and concerns regarding the surgery.
4. Changing the subject to divert the patient's attention from his anxiety.

Answer Key
The correct answer is 3.

Topic: Using Therapeutic Communication Techniques

The ability to use therapeutic communication techniques effectively is a crucial part of nursing and is highlighted in the NCLEX examination.

In the given question, the best response is option 3: "Encouraging the patient to talk about his feelings and concerns regarding the surgery." This technique is known as active listening, and it helps create a safe space for patients to express their fears and concerns. It validates the patient's feelings and allows the nurse to provide appropriate emotional support and information.

Option 1, giving advice, might be useful in some scenarios, but it's not the most appropriate approach in this case. It's more important for the nurse to listen to the patient's concerns and provide information to help them understand the situation better.

Option 2, telling the patient everything will be okay, is a form of false reassurance and is generally not recommended. It may dismiss the patient's feelings and concerns rather than addressing them effectively.

Option 4, changing the subject, is not an appropriate technique in this scenario. It could be seen as dismissive and might leave the patient feeling unheard or isolated with his anxiety.

In preparation for the NCLEX exam, understand that therapeutic communication techniques are a key aspect of patient care. These techniques help nurses understand and empathize with their patients, build trust, and provide appropriate emotional support. They form the basis of patient-centered care and can significantly improve patient outcomes.

Question 72

A psychiatric nurse is taking care of a client with severe anxiety. Which of the following actions would be most appropriate for promoting a therapeutic environment for this client?

1. Keeping the television on in the client's room to provide a distraction.
2. Providing a quiet, calm, and well-lit environment for the client.
3. Discussing the client's condition in detail with the other clients on the ward.
4. Frequently changing the client's room to give them a new environment.

Answer Key
The correct answer is 2.

Topic: Promoting a Therapeutic Environment

A therapeutic environment is critical to promoting healing, reducing stress, and increasing the comfort and well-being of clients. It encompasses both physical and psychological elements.

In the context of the NCLEX, a significant portion of questions related to promoting a therapeutic environment involve determining the nurse's best action in various scenarios. As such, a strong understanding of environmental factors and the impact on patient care is vital.

Option 2 is the best choice. Providing a quiet, calm, and well-lit environment can greatly reduce anxiety levels in clients. Such an environment can provide a sense of safety and predictability, helping the client feel more at ease.

Option 1, keeping the television on as a distraction, might not be effective for all clients. For some, it might indeed serve as a distraction, but for others, it can lead to sensory overload, especially in clients with anxiety disorders.

Option 3, discussing the client's condition with other clients, is inappropriate and breaches confidentiality laws. Always maintain the privacy and confidentiality of client information unless there's an informed consent or legal obligation to disclose.

Option 4, frequently changing the client's room, can be disruptive and increase anxiety rather than decrease it. Stability and familiarity of surroundings often aid in reducing anxiety.

When preparing for the NCLEX, remember to consider both the physical and psychological aspects of the environment. A quiet, calm, and consistent environment, along with a respectful and understanding approach from healthcare professionals, forms the basis of a therapeutic environment.

Question 73

A nurse is caring for a client who is hard of hearing. Which of the following interventions is MOST appropriate when communicating with this client?

1. Speak louder and faster to ensure the client hears the message.
2. Use a normal tone of voice and speak directly facing the client.
3. Write all communication on paper because verbal communication will not be effective.
4. Only communicate with the client when absolutely necessary to reduce frustration.

Answer Key
The correct answer is 2.

Topic: Assisting Clients with Physical or Sensory Impairments

Assisting clients with physical or sensory impairments is an essential aspect of nursing care. It involves both understanding the specific needs associated with the impairment and implementing effective strategies to optimize communication and overall care.

In this question, the client has a hearing impairment. The most effective communication strategy is option 2: using a normal tone of voice and speaking directly facing the client. This approach allows the client to use visual cues like lip reading and facial expressions to aid in understanding the conversation. Also, speaking clearly and at a moderate pace can facilitate comprehension.

Option 1, speaking louder and faster, can distort the words and make lip reading more difficult. It could also come across as aggressive or disrespectful.

Option 3, writing all communication, could be useful in some cases. However, it shouldn't be the only form of communication used, as it's time-consuming and may be impractical during a rapidly evolving situation. Also, not all clients may be able to read well.

Option 4, only communicating when absolutely necessary, is inappropriate. Effective and ongoing communication is crucial to provide high-quality care and to build trust with the client.

In the NCLEX exam, understanding the specific needs and best practices related to various physical and sensory impairments is important. Remember, the goal is to promote the independence, comfort, and safety of the client while ensuring effective communication and high-quality care.

Question 74

A client with a new ileostomy expresses concern about having to manage it at home. Which of the following responses from the nurse is MOST appropriate?

1. "Don't worry, with time everything becomes easier."
2. "I understand your concerns. Let's go through the process step by step."
3. "You should hire a home health aide to manage your ileostomy."
4. "There's no need for concern. It's not a complicated process."

Answer Key
The correct answer is 2.

Topic: Management of Bowel and Bladder Alteration

Management of bowel and bladder alterations is a key part of nursing care, especially for individuals who have undergone surgeries such as ileostomy. Understanding how to provide the appropriate education and emotional support is paramount.

In this question, the client expresses concern about managing their new ileostomy at home. The nurse's best response is option 2: acknowledging the client's concerns and providing education about the process. The nurse should reassure the client and demonstrate each step of the process, allowing the client to practice under supervision until they feel comfortable managing it independently.

Option 1, dismissing the client's worries, can make them feel unheard and unsupported, which is counterproductive to the establishment of trust.

Option 3, suggesting a home health aide, may not be feasible or desirable for the client and doesn't encourage the client's self-care and independence.

Option 4, diminishing the client's concerns, does not acknowledge the client's feelings of anxiety and fear.

In the NCLEX exam, questions on this topic often require knowledge of how to educate clients about self-care and how to provide emotional support. This involves understanding the procedures and practices associated with managing different bowel and bladder alterations and knowing how to communicate this information effectively to the client. Remember, every client's response to their alterations is individual and should be met with empathy, patience, and tailored education.

Question 75

A nurse is teaching a client how to perform a colostomy irrigation. Which of the following steps should be included in the teaching?

1. The client should lie flat while performing the irrigation.
2. The client should use warm water for the irrigation.
3. The irrigation bag should be held 3 feet above the stoma.
4. The client should insert the catheter 3 inches into the stoma.

Answer Key
The correct answer is 2.

Topic: Performing Irrigations

Colostomy irrigation is a method to regulate bowel movements by emptying the colon at a scheduled time. This procedure is not suitable for all clients with a colostomy but can provide more predictability and control for some. In the NCLEX exam, nurses must be familiar with how to teach this procedure to clients.

Option 1 is incorrect; the client should be sitting up, not lying flat. This position facilitates gravity flow of the solution into the colon.

Option 2 is correct; the client should use warm water for the irrigation to promote comfort and avoid cramping.

Option 3 is incorrect; the irrigation bag should be held at the level of the client's hip or approximately 18 inches above the stoma, not 3 feet. Holding it too high could increase the speed and pressure of the flow, leading to discomfort or damage.

Option 4 is incorrect; the catheter is inserted about 1 inch into the stoma, not 3 inches. Excessive insertion could damage the stoma or the underlying bowel.

Questions about this topic in the NCLEX exam may require nurses to apply their knowledge of anatomy, pathophysiology, and nursing procedures. It is essential to understand the proper steps in performing irrigations and how to teach these to clients to promote self-care and independence. Always prioritize client safety and comfort in all nursing procedures.

Question 76

A nurse is developing a plan of care for a bedridden client at risk for developing pressure ulcers. Which of the following interventions should be included in the plan?

1. Reposition the client every 4 hours.
2. Use a donut cushion for sitting.
3. Implement a high-protein diet.
4. Keep the head of the bed elevated at all times.

Answer Key
The correct answer is 3.

Topic: Skin Integrity Maintenance

Skin integrity maintenance, especially in bedridden clients, is a crucial aspect of nursing care. Pressure ulcers are a significant concern and can lead to severe complications if not prevented or treated promptly.

Option 1 is incorrect; a bedridden client at risk for pressure ulcers should be repositioned at least every 2 hours, not 4 hours. Prolonged pressure on a specific area increases the risk of skin breakdown.

Option 2 is incorrect; a donut cushion can lead to uneven pressure distribution, leading to a higher risk for pressure ulcers. Instead, a pressure-redistributing cushion should be used.

Option 3 is correct; a high-protein diet supports skin health and integrity and promotes healing. Ensuring the client receives adequate nutrition is an essential part of preventative care.

Option 4 is incorrect; the head of the bed should be kept at the lowest degree of elevation possible to prevent shear and friction, which can contribute to skin breakdown.

For NCLEX, understanding how to prevent and manage pressure ulcers is crucial. Candidates should be familiar with risk factors, preventative measures, and treatment options, as well as the importance of frequent skin assessments for at-risk clients. Skin integrity management requires a comprehensive approach that involves regular repositioning, pressure redistribution, proper nutrition, and good skincare.

Question 77

A nurse is teaching a client who recently had a leg amputation about using crutches. Which of the following statements by the client indicates a need for further instruction?

1. "I will place the crutches slightly in front of me before I step forward."
2. "I will put all my weight on my hands when using the crutches."
3. "I will avoid walking on slippery surfaces to prevent falls."
4. "I will inspect my armpits daily for any skin breakdown."

Answer Key
The correct answer is 2.

Topic: Orthopedic Devices Application and Maintenance

Understanding the proper use and maintenance of orthopedic devices is an important aspect of nursing care, especially for clients who have had limb amputations or who have impaired mobility.

Option 1 is correct; placing the crutches slightly ahead before stepping forward provides stability and balance.

Option 2 is incorrect; putting all the weight on the hands can lead to nerve damage in the hands and wrists. Instead, the body's weight should be supported by the arms and shoulders, not the hands.

Option 3 is correct; avoiding slippery surfaces is a good safety measure to prevent accidents and falls.

Option 4 is correct; frequent inspection of areas where the crutches come into contact with the skin (such as the armpits) is important to identify any signs of skin breakdown early.

For the NCLEX, it is crucial to understand the safety measures related to the use of orthopedic devices. Candidates should be familiar with the correct methods of using these devices and the common problems associated with their use, such as skin breakdown and nerve damage. Proper education of clients about the safe and effective use of these devices, as well as regular inspection and maintenance, are vital aspects of nursing care.

Question 78

A nurse is caring for a patient who is on bed rest after a major surgery. Which of the following interventions is most appropriate for the nurse to implement to promote circulation in this patient?

1. Massaging the patient's legs.
2. Encouraging the patient to perform leg and ankle exercises.
3. Placing a pillow under the patient's knees when lying down.
4. Keeping the patient in a supine position at all times.

Answer Key
The correct answer is 2.

Topic: Measures to Promote Circulation

Promoting circulation in patients, especially those on bed rest or with limited mobility, is a vital nursing responsibility. Proper circulation helps prevent the development of deep vein thrombosis, a potentially life-threatening complication.

Option 1 is incorrect; massaging the patient's legs, especially if they're at risk for or have a thrombus, can dislodge the clot leading to a pulmonary embolism.

Option 2 is correct; encouraging the patient to perform leg and ankle exercises promotes blood flow, reduces the risk of clot formation, and can improve overall cardiovascular health.

Option 3 is incorrect; placing a pillow under the patient's knees may limit blood flow and promote clot formation. The patient's legs should be in a neutral or dependent position.

Option 4 is incorrect; keeping the patient in a supine position at all times does not encourage circulation. Patients should be encouraged to change positions frequently.

For the NCLEX, understanding measures to promote circulation and prevent complications is crucial. It's important to know how to instruct patients on performing leg and ankle exercises, understanding the risks of massage or constant positions, and the importance of frequent position changes.

Question 79

A nurse is caring for a postoperative patient who is experiencing pain. Which of the following assessment is most appropriate for the nurse to utilize to gain objective data about the patient's pain?

1. Ask the patient about the location of the pain.
2. Observe the patient's facial expressions.
3. Use a pain scale to rate the severity of the pain.
4. Ask the patient about the quality of the pain.

Answer Key
The correct answer is 2.

Topic: Pain Assessment and Intervention

Pain assessment is a critical aspect of nursing care. It's important to utilize both subjective and objective data when assessing a patient's pain.

Option 1 is incorrect; asking the patient about the location of the pain provides subjective data because it comes directly from the patient's personal experience and perspective.

Option 2 is correct; observing the patient's facial expressions can provide objective data. Facial expressions like grimacing or wincing can indicate the presence of pain.

Option 3 is incorrect; using a pain scale to rate the severity of the pain provides subjective data as it's based on the patient's personal perception of the pain intensity.

Option 4 is incorrect; asking the patient about the quality of the pain (e.g., sharp, dull, burning) provides subjective data as it depends on the patient's personal experience of the pain.

When preparing for the NCLEX, it's vital to understand how to differentiate between subjective and objective data in pain assessment. Remember, objective data can be observed or measured, whereas subjective data are based on the patient's personal experiences and perceptions. An effective pain assessment and intervention strategy involves both types of data to provide comprehensive care.

Question 80

A patient who suffers from chronic lower back pain expresses interest in exploring complementary therapies. Which of the following options should the nurse suggest as potentially beneficial?

1. Massage therapy
2. Physical therapy
3. Acupuncture
4. All of the above

Answer Key
The correct answer is 4.

Topic: Evidence-based Complementary Therapies for Pain Management

Complementary therapies often play a crucial role in managing chronic pain when used alongside conventional medical treatments. Each option given in this question represents an evidence-based form of complementary therapy.

Option 1, Massage therapy, involves manipulating the body's muscles and soft tissues to relieve pain and tension. It's been found to be effective in reducing pain and improving function in people with chronic lower back pain.

Option 2, Physical therapy, often includes exercises to improve mobility and strength, as well as techniques to manage pain. It is widely accepted and proven to be beneficial in managing chronic lower back pain, helping to improve mobility, strength, and overall quality of life.

Option 3, Acupuncture, a practice in traditional Chinese medicine, involves inserting thin needles into specific points on the body. Studies have shown it to be potentially beneficial for chronic lower back pain, and it's recommended by some guidelines for this condition.

When preparing for the NCLEX, it's important to understand the role of evidence-based complementary therapies in pain management. Nurses should have an understanding of various therapies, their potential benefits, and their appropriateness for different patients and situations. Knowing these therapies and how to incorporate them into patient care plans can significantly enhance the quality of care.

Question 81

A nurse is caring for a patient who has had a recent left-sided stroke and is having trouble swallowing. Which position would be most appropriate for this patient during meal times?

1. Supine position
2. Trendelenburg position
3. High Fowler's position
4. Prone position

Answer Key

The correct answer is 3.

Topic: Positioning for Comfort and Safety

In the nursing profession, positioning patients appropriately is crucial not only for their comfort but also for their safety. Each of the positions listed above serves a specific purpose, but not all are suitable for every patient.

Option 1, the Supine position, in which the patient lies flat on their back, is not ideal in this situation as it could increase the risk of aspiration (food or fluid entering the windpipe and lungs).

Option 2, the Trendelenburg position, in which the body is laid flat on the back (supine position) with the feet higher than the head by 15-30 degrees, is typically used for shock or certain surgeries, but not for patients with swallowing difficulties.

Option 3, the High Fowler's position, in which the patient is sitting up at an angle between 60-90 degrees, is the most appropriate choice in this scenario. This position can help to reduce the risk of aspiration during meals by using gravity to help keep food and fluids moving downward during swallowing.

Option 4, the Prone position, where the patient lies flat on their stomach, is not suitable for meal times.

Remember, when it comes to the NCLEX, safety is a priority. Knowing how to position patients based on their specific needs and health status is an essential aspect of providing safe and effective care. Always prioritize patient comfort, safety, and the prevention of potential complications when determining appropriate positioning.

Question 82

A nurse is preparing to assist with a lumbar puncture for a patient suspected of having bacterial meningitis. Which of the following actions is the most appropriate for the nurse to take?

1. Place the patient in a supine position with their legs extended.
2. Administer a muscle relaxant prior to the procedure.
3. Instruct the patient to hold their breath during needle insertion.
4. Position the patient in lateral recumbent position with their knees drawn up to the chest.

Answer Key
The correct answer is 4.

Topic: Assisting with Invasive Procedures

When assisting with invasive procedures, it's critical for nurses to understand the specific patient positioning and pre-procedural requirements for each procedure. A lumbar puncture, often referred to as a spinal tap, is a procedure used to collect a sample of cerebrospinal fluid for diagnostic purposes.

In the options provided:
1. Placing the patient in a supine position with their legs extended is incorrect. This position would not allow for the optimal exposure of the lumbar region of the spine, where the needle needs to be inserted.
2. Administering a muscle relaxant is not typically part of the protocol for a lumbar puncture. The procedure requires patient cooperation, and a muscle relaxant might inhibit this.
3. Instructing the patient to hold their breath during needle insertion is incorrect. Patients are generally advised to relax and breathe normally during the procedure to prevent any unnecessary movement.
4. Positioning the patient in the lateral recumbent position (on their side) with their knees drawn up to their chest is the most appropriate action. This position helps to open up the spaces between the

vertebrae in the lower back, allowing for easier and safer needle insertion.

Remember, as a nurse assisting with invasive procedures, it's not only your role to understand the procedure's requirements but also to ensure the patient's comfort, safety, and understanding of what is going to occur. This reduces anxiety and promotes cooperation, which can lead to better outcomes. The NCLEX will test your understanding of these essential aspects of patient care.

Question 83

A nurse is caring for a newborn undergoing phototherapy for neonatal jaundice. Which of the following interventions should the nurse perform?

1. Cover the newborn's eyes with protective patches.
2. Apply lotion to the newborn's skin to prevent dryness.
3. Keep the newborn clothed to prevent hypothermia.
4. Increase feedings to promote bilirubin excretion.

Answer Key
The correct answer is 1.

Topic: Implementing and Monitoring Phototherapy

Phototherapy is a common treatment for neonatal jaundice, a condition that results from high levels of bilirubin in a newborn's blood. The treatment involves shining fluorescent light on the baby's skin, which changes the shape and structure of the bilirubin molecules, enabling them to be excreted in the baby's urine and stools.

Let's analyze the options:
1. Covering the newborn's eyes with protective patches is correct. The intense light used during phototherapy can harm the baby's sensitive eyes, so they must be shielded.
2. Applying lotion to the newborn's skin is not recommended during phototherapy. It could potentially interfere with the effectiveness of the treatment by blocking the light and creating a barrier on the skin.
3. Keeping the newborn clothed can interfere with the treatment as it blocks the light from reaching the baby's skin. In phototherapy, the newborn is usually undressed to allow maximum skin exposure to the light, but the genital area is covered.
4. While frequent feeding does help in promoting bilirubin excretion, it's not directly related to the

phototherapy process. Hence, increasing feedings is not the most appropriate action in this case.

Question 84

A nurse is caring for an older adult patient who is at risk of hypothermia due to decreased thermoregulation. Which of the following interventions should the nurse implement to maintain the patient's optimal body temperature?

1. Encourage the patient to engage in regular physical activity.
2. Limit the use of blankets and warm clothing.
3. Provide warm, non-caffeinated beverages.
4. Apply cold compresses periodically.

Answer Key
The correct answer is 3.

Topic: Maintaining Optimal Temperature of Client

In nursing practice, maintaining the optimal body temperature of clients, especially those who are vulnerable, such as older adults, is crucial. Age can impact the body's ability to regulate temperature, making older adults more susceptible to hypothermia in cold environments.

Let's discuss the options:
1. Regular physical activity can help generate heat in the body. However, in an older adult who is already at risk of hypothermia, physical activity might not be the best or most immediate solution to maintain body temperature.
2. Limiting the use of blankets and warm clothing is incorrect. These items help to conserve body heat and should be utilized as necessary to keep an at-risk patient warm.
3. Providing warm, non-caffeinated beverages is the correct choice. Warm beverages can help raise body temperature from the inside, while avoiding caffeine helps prevent increased urine output, which could lead to more heat loss.
4. Applying cold compresses would further decrease body temperature, which is not the desired outcome for a patient at risk of hypothermia.

To prepare for the NCLEX exam on this topic, understand the importance of temperature regulation and the interventions that can help maintain body temperature. Knowledge of how to prevent, identify, and treat temperature-related conditions like hypothermia and hyperthermia is vital. Additionally, understanding the different factors that can influence a client's ability to regulate body temperature (like age, certain diseases, and certain medications) can inform your nursing interventions.

Question 85

A nurse is caring for a client on a ventilator. Which of the following actions should the nurse take to provide the best care for this client?

1. Limit oral care to prevent any discomfort.
2. Place the client in a supine position to promote lung expansion.
3. Conduct frequent respiratory assessments.
4. Reduce sedation to allow the client to breathe on their own.

Answer Key
The correct answer is 3.

Topic: Monitoring and Caring for Clients on a Ventilator

Monitoring and caring for clients on a ventilator is a critical aspect of nursing care, particularly in intensive care units. Ventilators support breathing in patients who are unable to breathe adequately on their own, often because of acute illness, surgery, or injury.

Let's explore each option:
1. Limiting oral care is incorrect. Regular oral care is critical in ventilated patients as it helps reduce the risk of ventilator-associated pneumonia.
2. Placing the client in a supine position is incorrect. This position can actually decrease lung expansion and promote atelectasis and pneumonia. A semi-upright position is recommended for ventilated patients when feasible.
3. Conducting frequent respiratory assessments is the correct choice. It's crucial to monitor the client's respiratory status, ventilator settings, and response to the mechanical ventilation frequently. Changes in lung sounds, oxygen saturation, and other respiratory parameters can indicate potential problems like pneumothorax or deterioration in the patient's condition.

4. Reducing sedation is not always appropriate and should be based on the client's condition and the doctor's orders. While minimizing sedation can be part of a ventilator weaning process, it should be done under careful monitoring and assessment.

When preparing for the NCLEX exam on this topic, focus on understanding the purpose of mechanical ventilation, the nursing responsibilities associated with ventilator care, and potential complications. Knowledge of ventilator settings, modes, and alarms, as well as interventions to prevent complications, such as oral care and patient positioning, are also crucial. A comprehensive understanding of respiratory assessment is key to providing safe and effective care to a patient on a ventilator.

Question 86

A nurse is caring for a patient who just had a surgical procedure and has a newly placed drainage system. Which of the following actions should the nurse take to ensure proper monitoring and maintenance of the drainage system?

1. Empty the drainage container every 24 hours.
2. Ensure the drainage system is hanging above the patient's surgical site.
3. Document the amount, color, and consistency of the drainage.
4. Discourage the patient from moving to avoid disrupting the drainage system.

Answer Key
The correct answer is 3.

Topic: Drainage Device Monitoring and Maintenance

Drainage systems are often used after surgical procedures to remove fluid buildup, reducing the risk of infection or complications. It's crucial for nurses to understand how to monitor and maintain these devices properly.

Let's explore each option:
1. Emptying the drainage container every 24 hours is not always accurate. Depending on the type of drain and the rate of drainage, it may need to be emptied more often. The nurse must empty the container when it is filled to the manufacturer's recommendation, usually halfway or two-thirds full.
2. Ensuring the drainage system is hanging above the patient's surgical site is incorrect. Drainage systems should be kept below the level of the surgical site to promote gravity flow of drainage.
3. Documenting the amount, color, and consistency of the drainage is correct. This allows for accurate monitoring of the patient's healing progress and early detection of complications such as infection or hemorrhage. Unexpected changes should be reported promptly.
4. Discouraging the patient from moving is incorrect. While care should be taken not to disrupt the drain,

mobility is essential for patient recovery. Nurses should educate patients on how to move safely without dislodging the drain.

The NCLEX exam requires a good understanding of the different types of drainage systems, including Jackson-Pratt drains, Hemovac drains, and chest tubes. This knowledge includes how to monitor for complications, how often to empty the drains, and how to maintain the device's integrity. Reviewing the signs of potential issues, such as signs of infection or drain dislodgement, is also critical. With thorough knowledge and application of these principles, nurses can ensure patient safety and promote healing.

Question 87

A nurse is providing care for a client who is undergoing peritoneal dialysis. Which of the following interventions should the nurse prioritize?

1. Advising the client to restrict fluid intake during treatment.
2. Observing the color and clarity of the dialysate outflow.
3. Administering intravenous antibiotics prophylactically.
4. Monitoring the client's serum glucose levels only before the procedure.

Answer Key
The correct answer is 2.

Topic: Peritoneal Dialysis Performance and Management

Peritoneal dialysis is a treatment that uses the lining of your abdomen, or belly, to filter your blood. It's a complex process requiring careful oversight from nursing professionals, with distinct considerations for patient safety and wellbeing.

Let's break down each option:
1. Advising the client to restrict fluid intake during treatment may not always be the best intervention. The client's fluid needs vary depending on several factors, such as the client's residual kidney function and the amount of urine output. The fluid restriction may be necessary for some, but not all clients.
2. Observing the color and clarity of the dialysate outflow is a key nursing responsibility. The fluid should be clear or slightly yellow. Cloudy dialysate, or the presence of fibrin or blood, could indicate complications like infection or catheter malposition.
3. Administering intravenous antibiotics prophylactically is not a standard practice in peritoneal dialysis unless there's a specific reason for it, such as a recent infection.
4. Monitoring the client's serum glucose levels only before the procedure is not adequate. Dialysate

contains dextrose, which can cause increased blood glucose levels, so regular monitoring is crucial during the procedure, not just before.

For the NCLEX, it's critical to remember that peritoneal dialysis is not without risks, and the nurse should know how to monitor for signs of infection, ensure the safe and effective performance of the procedure, and provide comprehensive care and education to the client. This includes understanding the principles of aseptic technique when caring for the dialysis catheter and recognizing the signs and symptoms of peritonitis. Furthermore, understanding the principles of fluid balance and electrolyte management, along with potential complications of the procedure, is crucial. Reviewing these elements in-depth will equip you with the necessary knowledge to navigate this topic effectively in the exam.

Question 88

A nurse is preparing to suction a client with a tracheostomy. Which of the following actions should the nurse perform first?

1. Apply suction while withdrawing the catheter.
2. Assess the client's oxygen saturation levels.
3. Lubricate the suction catheter with sterile saline.
4. Use sterile gloves to handle the suction catheter.

Answer Key
The correct answer is 2.

Topic: Performing Suctioning

Suctioning is a critical procedure that is performed to maintain a patent airway and prevent respiratory distress in patients with artificial airways such as tracheostomies or endotracheal tubes.

Let's break down each option:
1. Applying suction while withdrawing the catheter is a correct action during the procedure, but it's not the first thing a nurse should do.
2. Assessing the client's oxygen saturation levels is the first action a nurse should take before suctioning. It provides a baseline for the patient's oxygenation status and allows the nurse to ensure the client is stable enough to withstand the procedure. It's crucial to understand that suctioning can cause hypoxia and may lead to a drop in oxygen saturation levels.
3. Lubricating the suction catheter with sterile saline is a part of the procedure, but it isn't the initial step.
4. Using sterile gloves to handle the suction catheter is an essential component of maintaining asepsis during the procedure, but it comes after initial patient assessment.

For the NCLEX exam, remember that suctioning is an invasive procedure that requires strict adherence to sterile technique and careful assessment of the patient before, during, and after the procedure. It's important to understand the risks involved with suctioning, including hypoxia, trauma to the airway, infection, and cardiac dysrhythmias. Furthermore, understanding when suctioning is necessary (such as visible secretions, adventitious lung sounds, increased respiratory distress, or decreased oxygen saturation) is a key part of providing safe and effective care. Thoroughly reviewing these principles will help ensure your preparedness for any suctioning-related questions on the NCLEX exam.

Question 89

A nurse is preparing to change a client's surgical wound dressing. Which of the following steps should be taken first?

1. Gather necessary supplies.
2. Apply sterile gloves.
3. Perform hand hygiene.
4. Remove the old dressing.

Answer Key
The correct answer is 3.

Topic: Wound Care and Dressing Change

Wound care and dressing changes are fundamental skills in nursing. The goal is to promote wound healing, prevent infection, and maintain healthy skin integrity.

Let's analyze each option:
1. Gathering necessary supplies is an important step in the process of changing a wound dressing, but it's not the first one.
2. Applying sterile gloves is a crucial part of maintaining asepsis during the procedure, but it is not the first step.
3. Performing hand hygiene is the first and most essential step before any clinical procedure. It is a simple, cost-effective method for preventing the spread of pathogenic microorganisms and reducing the incidence of health care-associated infections.
4. Removing the old dressing is part of the procedure, but it comes after hand hygiene, gathering supplies, and applying gloves.

In preparation for the NCLEX, it's important to understand not only the process of wound care and dressing changes but also the principles behind them. These include maintaining aseptic technique, understanding the stages of wound healing, knowing the different types of wound dressings, and being able to identify signs of infection or complications. Additionally, providing appropriate client education about wound care, including the importance of nutrition and hydration, is key. Lastly, remember to provide comfort measures, as dressing changes can sometimes be uncomfortable or painful for clients. Understanding these aspects will help you answer questions about wound care on the NCLEX accurately.

Question 90

A nurse is providing education to a client who recently had an ileostomy. Which of the following statements by the client indicates a need for further teaching?

1. "I should change my ostomy pouch when it's about one-third full."
2. "I can expect my ostomy output to be liquid to semi-formed."
3. "I can eat a normal diet after six to eight weeks post-surgery."
4. "I should only clean the skin around my stoma with alcohol."

Answer Key
The correct answer is 4.

Topic: Providing Ostomy Care and Education

Ostomy care and education is a crucial part of nursing, especially for clients who have recently undergone an ostomy surgery. This procedure can drastically change a person's life, and they often rely heavily on their healthcare providers for information and support.

Let's analyze each option:
1. Changing the ostomy pouch when it's about one-third full is correct. Waiting until the pouch is fuller could lead to leaks or even damage the skin around the stoma.
2. Expecting the ostomy output to be liquid to semi-formed is correct. The consistency of the output depends on the location of the ostomy. In the case of an ileostomy, because the waste has not reached the colon where most of the water is absorbed, it is usually liquid to semi-formed.
3. The statement about being able to eat a normal diet after six to eight weeks post-surgery is also correct. However, clients are often advised to start with a low-residue diet and gradually reintroduce other foods while observing how their body reacts.
4. The client should not clean the skin around the stoma with alcohol. This can dry out and irritate the skin. Instead, warm water and a soft cloth should be used.

In preparation for the NCLEX, remember that proper ostomy care involves maintaining skin integrity, monitoring for complications, managing the appliance, and providing emotional support and education to the client. Key areas for patient education include hygiene, diet, activity, and self-care, including how to change the ostomy bag, monitor for skin irritation or infection, and notice signs of obstruction or dehydration. Each client's situation is unique, so it's important to tailor education to their specific needs.

Question 91

A nurse is caring for a client with chronic obstructive pulmonary disease (COPD). Which of the following interventions would be the most effective in promoting pulmonary hygiene for this client?

1. Encourage deep breathing exercises every 4 hours.
2. Administer prescribed bronchodilators before chest physiotherapy.
3. Keep the client in a supine position as much as possible.
4. Limit fluid intake to prevent fluid overload.

Answer Key
The correct answer is 2.

Topic: Providing Pulmonary Hygiene

Pulmonary hygiene, also known as bronchial or lung hygiene, involves methods used to clear mucus and secretions from the lungs. This is particularly important in clients with respiratory diseases like COPD, where there's an excess production of mucus that can block the airways and cause breathing difficulties.

Here's a breakdown of the answer choices:
1. Encouraging deep breathing exercises is beneficial for all clients, especially those with respiratory diseases. However, for a client with COPD, simply encouraging deep breathing exercises every 4 hours might not be sufficient for effective pulmonary hygiene.
2. Administering prescribed bronchodilators before chest physiotherapy is the correct answer. Bronchodilators help to open up the airways, making it easier for chest physiotherapy to mobilize secretions.
3. Keeping the client in a supine position as much as possible is incorrect. A semi-upright position, like Fowler's position, can enhance lung expansion and help in secretion clearance.
4. Limiting fluid intake to prevent fluid overload is not generally recommended unless the client has a specific condition like heart failure. For most COPD

patients, adequate hydration helps thin out mucus, making it easier to clear from the airways.

As a nurse preparing for the NCLEX, understanding the purpose and implementation of pulmonary hygiene techniques is crucial. Techniques like chest physiotherapy, percussion, postural drainage, vibration, effective coughing, deep breathing exercises, and the use of bronchodilators can all play a part in pulmonary hygiene. Patient education about the importance of these interventions, as well as lifestyle modifications such as smoking cessation, can significantly improve the client's respiratory status.

Question 92

A nurse is caring for a client who has just returned from the recovery room after undergoing a cholecystectomy. What should be the nurse's priority action?

1. Assess the client's level of consciousness.
2. Check the client's vital signs.
3. Inspect the surgical dressing for signs of bleeding.
4. Assist the client in performing leg exercises.

Answer Key
The correct answer is 2.

Topic: Postoperative Care Provision

Postoperative care provision involves a range of nursing interventions aimed at monitoring and managing the client's condition after surgery. The initial period after surgery is critical as it's the time when the client is most vulnerable to complications such as hemorrhage, hypovolemic shock, thromboembolism, infection, and respiratory issues like atelectasis and pneumonia.

Let's break down the options:
1. Assessing the client's level of consciousness is important but isn't usually the priority action in immediate postoperative care unless the client underwent neurosurgery or there's a suspicion of brain-related complications.
2. Checking the client's vital signs is the priority action in immediate postoperative care. Vital signs include blood pressure, pulse, respiration rate, temperature, and oxygen saturation. These provide critical information about the client's cardiovascular and respiratory status, helping the nurse detect early signs of complications such as bleeding, shock, or respiratory distress.
3. Inspecting the surgical dressing for signs of bleeding is a crucial part of postoperative care, but it isn't typically the first action. After checking the vital signs,

the nurse can then focus on the surgical site and other specific aspects of care.
4. Assisting the client in performing leg exercises is an essential part of preventing deep vein thrombosis (DVT) in postoperative clients. However, this wouldn't be the priority in the immediate postoperative period.

As an NCLEX candidate, it's important to understand the priorities in postoperative care provision. These include monitoring vital signs, observing for signs of complications, managing pain, encouraging mobility, providing wound care, and promoting effective breathing and coughing.

Remember, the goal of postoperative care is to aid recovery, prevent complications, and promote the client's return to their baseline health status. Key factors to consider in postoperative care include the type of surgery, the client's overall health status, the anesthesia used, and the client's response to the surgery. Understanding these elements will enable you to provide comprehensive, tailored care to meet the unique needs of each postoperative client.

Question 93

A nurse is caring for a client with severe diarrhea. Which of the following symptoms would the nurse anticipate as a potential indication of hypokalemia?

1. Hyperreflexia.
2. Flushed, dry skin.
3. Muscle weakness.
4. Bradycardia.

Answer Key
The correct answer is 3.

Topic: Fluid and Electrolyte Imbalance Management

Fluid and electrolyte balance is crucial in maintaining homeostasis within the body. Electrolytes, including potassium, sodium, calcium, magnesium, bicarbonate, phosphate, and chloride, have numerous physiological roles. They assist in maintaining fluid balance, contribute to nerve impulse transmission and muscle contraction, help regulate the body's acid-base balance, and support cellular function.

In this question, we're considering hypokalemia, which is a lower-than-normal amount of potassium in the blood. Potassium is vital for cell metabolism, cardiac function, nerve impulse transmission, and muscle contraction.

When managing a client with a potential fluid and electrolyte imbalance like diarrhea, the nurse needs to monitor electrolyte levels, assess for symptoms of imbalance, administer prescribed treatments, and provide appropriate client education.

Looking at the options:
1. Hyperreflexia is more typically associated with hyperkalemia (high potassium), not hypokalemia.
2. Flushed, dry skin is commonly seen in dehydration or hyperthermia, not specifically in hypokalemia.

3. Muscle weakness is a key symptom of hypokalemia. Potassium plays a crucial role in muscle cell function, so when levels are low, muscle weakness, cramping, or even paralysis can occur.
4. Bradycardia can be a symptom of hyperkalemia, not hypokalemia. Hypokalemia typically presents with tachycardia.

Understanding electrolyte imbalances is a crucial component of the NCLEX exam. For example, imbalances like hypokalemia and hyperkalemia are serious conditions that can significantly affect the heart's rhythm, leading to life-threatening arrhythmias. Other symptoms can include changes in muscle function, nerve transmission, mental status, and other physiological processes.

Treatment of electrolyte imbalances involves addressing the underlying cause, administering supplements or medications as necessary, and educating the client about the importance of diet in maintaining balance. In the case of hypokalemia, treatment might include oral or intravenous potassium supplementation and dietary modifications to include potassium-rich foods like bananas, oranges, and leafy greens.

As an NCLEX candidate, you should familiarize yourself with the various electrolytes, their normal values, their roles in the body, the causes and symptoms of their imbalances, and how to manage these imbalances. Also, understand how to interpret laboratory results and how to monitor clients for potential complications. You should also be able to educate clients on dietary considerations related to maintaining proper electrolyte balance and when to seek medical help.

Question 94

A nurse is caring for a client with an arterial line (A-line). Which of the following actions is appropriate when caring for a client with an A-line?

1. Frequently reposition the client.
2. Use the line for routine blood draws.
3. Level the transducer at the phlebostatic axis.
4. Flush the line with 10 ml of heparin solution.

Answer Key

The correct answer is 3.

Topic: Arterial Line Monitoring and Maintenance

Arterial line (A-line) monitoring is an advanced hemodynamic monitoring method often used in critical care settings. An A-line allows for continuous blood pressure monitoring and easy arterial blood gas sampling. It's typically placed in the radial artery, although the femoral and brachial arteries can also be used.

Let's break down the options:

1. While it's generally good practice to reposition clients to prevent pressure ulcers, you must take extra care with A-line patients. Excessive movement can dislodge the catheter, potentially leading to complications such as hemorrhage or arterial occlusion.
2. Using the line for routine blood draws is one of the benefits of having an A-line. However, it should be done cautiously and according to facility policy as it could increase the risk of infection and other complications.
3. The transducer should be leveled at the phlebostatic axis (roughly at the level of the right atrium or fourth intercostal space at the mid-axillary line) to ensure accurate readings. This is a correct practice.
4. Flushing the A-line with 10 ml of heparin solution is incorrect. A-lines are usually flushed with a saline

solution, not heparin, to prevent clot formation. The amount and frequency of flushes would depend on the facility protocol.

As a nurse, the care for a client with an arterial line involves regular assessment and documentation of the insertion site for signs of infection or complications, ensuring the system is zeroed and calibrated accurately, and monitoring the arterial waveform for changes.

For the NCLEX, you should understand the purpose of an arterial line, the potential complications, and how to properly care for a patient with an A-line. Also, be aware of interventions to prevent those complications.

Remember, any abnormalities or changes in the client's condition should be reported promptly to the healthcare provider. Also, patient education about the purpose of the arterial line and any restrictions they need to follow to prevent complications is critical.

Question 95

A nurse is caring for a client who just had a pacemaker inserted. Which of the following instructions should the nurse provide to the client?

1. Avoid lifting your arm above your head on the side of the pacemaker.
2. It's normal for the pacemaker to cause a constant chest pain.
3. You can resume full physical activity immediately after the procedure.
4. MRI scans are safe as a pacemaker is made with non-magnetic material.

Answer Key
The correct answer is 1.

Topic: Pacing Device Care Management

Pacing devices, such as pacemakers and implantable cardioverter defibrillators (ICDs), are used to regulate heart rhythms. Management of these devices requires careful monitoring, patient education, and regular follow-up.

Reviewing the options:
1. Avoid lifting your arm above your head on the side of the pacemaker - This is correct. After insertion of a pacemaker, it is recommended that the client avoid lifting their arm above shoulder level on the side of the pacemaker to prevent lead displacement until the lead has had sufficient time to settle into the heart muscle (usually around 4-6 weeks post-insertion).
2. It's normal for the pacemaker to cause a constant chest pain - This is incorrect. Pain, discomfort, swelling, or redness at the generator site or changes in symptoms (e.g., increased dizziness, fainting, or palpitations) could indicate a problem with the pacemaker and should be reported immediately.
3. You can resume full physical activity immediately after the procedure - This is incorrect. Patients are generally advised to avoid strenuous physical activity for a period of time post-procedure to allow the pacemaker site to heal and to prevent lead displacement.

4. MRI scans are safe - This is incorrect. Although some newer pacemakers are MRI compatible, many are not, and MRI can potentially alter the function of the pacemaker or heat the leads. Patients should always consult their cardiologist before having an MRI.

As a candidate preparing for the NCLEX, you must understand the nursing management of patients with a pacing device. It involves monitoring for complications, promoting wound healing, providing patient education regarding activity restrictions, follow-up care, signs of infection or device malfunction, and when and how to seek help.

Furthermore, healthcare professionals should check the device's settings and function regularly, which often can be done remotely. Battery life also should be checked during follow-up visits. Battery depletion can lead to loss of pacing function, which could have serious consequences for the patient. Lastly, be aware of the potential for electromagnetic interference with pacing devices. Patients should be advised to keep cell phones and other devices that emit electromagnetic radiation away from their pacemaker.

Question 96

A nurse is caring for a client who is on a telemetry unit. Which of the following actions by the nurse is most important?

1. Use skin prep before attaching the telemetry electrodes.
2. Check the telemetry monitor for accurate reading every 8 hours.
3. Ignore artifact readings as these are normal with telemetry.
4. Position the electrodes on the right side of the chest for an accurate reading.

Answer Key
The correct answer is 1.

Topic: Telemetry Client Care Management

Telemetry is a tool that provides continuous monitoring of clients' heart rhythms and heart rates. It is commonly used in various hospital settings, especially in cardiac units. Nurses caring for clients on telemetry units need to understand the principles of its use and the management of patients using telemetry.

Breaking down the options:
1. Use skin prep before attaching the telemetry electrodes - Correct. Proper skin preparation ensures good electrode-skin contact, reducing artifact and ensuring accurate readings. This typically includes cleaning the skin with alcohol and possibly shaving excessive hair.
2. Check the telemetry monitor for accurate reading every 8 hours - Incorrect. The telemetry monitor should be checked more frequently than every 8 hours, as changes in a patient's heart rhythm can occur rapidly, and timely detection and intervention are crucial.
3. Ignore artifact readings as these are normal with telemetry - Incorrect. Artifacts, or "noise" in the telemetry readings, can interfere with the accurate interpretation of the cardiac rhythm. Nurses should

assess the client and reposition or replace electrodes if necessary to reduce artifact.
4. Position the electrodes on the right side of the chest for an accurate reading - Incorrect. Electrode placement varies, but usually, electrodes are placed on the left side of the chest to get the most accurate reading of the heart's electrical activity.

As a future NCLEX test taker, understanding the use and management of telemetry is crucial. Nurses have a responsibility to monitor the patient's heart rhythm regularly and take appropriate action in response to any detected abnormalities.

Additionally, it's also essential to educate the patient about the purpose of telemetry monitoring and the importance of notifying the nurse if they feel any discomfort, changes, or if the electrodes become loose. Lastly, nurses should be aware of potential interference sources with telemetry signals, including certain equipment and devices, and take steps to mitigate any interference.

Question 97

A nurse is caring for a client who is scheduled to receive hemodialysis today. Which of the following actions should the nurse prioritize?

1. Administer the client's prescribed antihypertensive medications.
2. Assess the client's vascular access site for signs of infection.
3. Provide a high-protein diet for the client before the procedure.
4. Encourage the client to drink water to stay hydrated.

Answer Key
The correct answer is 2.

Topic: Hemodialysis or Continuous Renal Replacement Therapy Care Management

Hemodialysis and Continuous Renal Replacement Therapy (CRRT) are common interventions for clients with kidney failure or acute kidney injury. They involve the removal of waste products and excess fluid from the blood when the kidneys cannot perform these tasks. The management of these clients is multifaceted and includes regular assessments, diet control, medication management, and education.

Breaking down the options:
1. Administer the client's prescribed antihypertensive medications - Incorrect. Generally, certain medications, such as antihypertensives, should be held prior to hemodialysis to avoid hypotension during the procedure.
2. Assess the client's vascular access site for signs of infection - Correct. This should be a priority. Infections can lead to serious complications like sepsis. Signs of infection can include redness, swelling, warmth, or pain at the access site.
3. Provide a high-protein diet for the client before the procedure - Incorrect. While clients on hemodialysis do require high-protein diets, meal timing should be coordinated around the dialysis schedule. A large

meal before dialysis may lead to nausea or hypotension during the procedure.
4. Encourage the client to drink water to stay hydrated - Incorrect. Fluid restrictions are generally necessary for clients on hemodialysis due to impaired kidney function.

For the NCLEX exam, understanding the needs of clients undergoing hemodialysis or CRRT is crucial. They require specialized care that involves collaboration between the client, the healthcare team, and often family members as well. Ensuring infection control, promoting dietary and fluid restrictions, and managing medications are key areas of focus. Also, client and family education about the process and what to expect, as well as signs of potential complications to report, is an important aspect of care. Regular psychosocial support may also be necessary, as the impact of chronic illness and the demands of treatment can be challenging.

Question 98

A nurse is caring for a client with a newly diagnosed Deep Vein Thrombosis (DVT). Which of the following interventions should the nurse prioritize?

1. Encouraging the client to exercise regularly.
2. Monitoring the client's partial thromboplastin time (PTT) levels.
3. Administering prescribed oral antibiotics.
4. Teaching the client to perform self-checks for skin cancer.

Answer Key
The correct answer is 2.

Topic: Care of Clients with Hemodynamic, Tissue Perfusion, and Hemostasis Alterations

The care of clients with alterations in hemodynamics, tissue perfusion, and hemostasis often involves managing conditions such as Deep Vein Thrombosis (DVT), which is characterized by the formation of a blood clot in the deep veins, typically in the legs. This condition can lead to serious complications like pulmonary embolism if the clot dislodges and travels to the lungs.

Breaking down the options:
1. Encouraging the client to exercise regularly - Incorrect. While mild exercise can be beneficial, it's essential to first confirm the appropriateness of this intervention with the healthcare provider to prevent dislodging the clot.
2. Monitoring the client's partial thromboplastin time (PTT) levels - Correct. Patients with DVT are often treated with anticoagulants to prevent the blood clot from getting bigger and to stop new clots from forming. The PTT test measures the time it takes for the blood to clot and is used to monitor the effectiveness of anticoagulant therapy.
3. Administering prescribed oral antibiotics - Incorrect. Antibiotics are used to treat bacterial infections, not DVT.

4. Teaching the client to perform self-checks for skin cancer - Incorrect. While skin checks are important, this is not a priority for a client with DVT.

For the NCLEX, remember that clients with DVT require careful monitoring and management. This includes anticoagulant therapy, regular lab testing such as PTT levels, and careful monitoring for signs of complications. Client education on recognizing signs of complications, such as chest pain, shortness of breath, and increased leg pain or swelling, is also essential. Understanding the complex needs of these clients will enhance your ability to provide safe, effective care and education.

Question 99

A nurse is educating a client recently diagnosed with Type 2 diabetes. What is the most important information the nurse should provide?

1. The benefits of a regular exercise regimen.
2. How to perform blood glucose monitoring.
3. Information about joining a local support group.
4. The importance of taking insulin as prescribed.

Answer Key
The correct answer is 2.

Topic: Education Regarding Acute or Chronic Conditions

Patient education is a critical part of managing acute and chronic conditions like diabetes. This not only empowers patients to participate actively in their care but also improves health outcomes and adherence to treatment plans.

Analyzing the options:
1. The benefits of a regular exercise regimen - Incorrect. While regular exercise is essential for managing diabetes, understanding how to monitor blood glucose levels is more critical as it directly impacts day-to-day management of the disease.
2. How to perform blood glucose monitoring - Correct. Monitoring blood glucose levels is vital for patients with diabetes as it informs them when their glucose levels are too high or too low, enabling timely intervention.
3. Information about joining a local support group - Incorrect. While emotional support can be beneficial, it is not as crucial as knowing how to manage blood glucose levels.
4. The importance of taking insulin as prescribed - Incorrect. While this is important for some people with diabetes, not all patients with Type 2 diabetes

require insulin. It's critical to tailor education to the individual patient's treatment regimen.

For the NCLEX, it's important to understand that patient education should be prioritized based on the patient's immediate needs and their ability to impact their health. For a patient with a new diagnosis of a chronic illness like diabetes, understanding how to manage their condition on a day-to-day basis, including monitoring blood glucose levels, dietary modifications, and medication management, is critical.

Question 100

A client with chronic obstructive pulmonary disease (COPD) experiences an increase in dyspnea. The nurse should prioritize which of the following interventions?

1. Encourage the client to use a pursed-lip breathing technique.
2. Administer a bronchodilator medication.
3. Position the client in a supine position.
4. Schedule respiratory therapy for the afternoon.

Answer Key
The correct answer is 1.

Topic: Management of Clients with Impaired Ventilation/Oxygenation

Nurses play a pivotal role in managing clients with impaired ventilation or oxygenation, such as those suffering from COPD. This management includes prompt recognition of symptoms, implementing interventions to improve oxygenation, administering medication, and educating patients about self-care techniques.

Examining the options:
1. Encourage the client to use a pursed-lip breathing technique - Correct. Pursed-lip breathing is a simple technique that improves ventilation, helps keep airways open longer, and promotes better gas exchange. It can help reduce dyspnea in patients with COPD.
2. Administer a bronchodilator medication - Incorrect. While bronchodilator medications are often used in COPD management, in this scenario, the nurse needs to first utilize non-pharmacological measures like the pursed-lip breathing technique.
3. Position the client in a supine position - Incorrect. The supine position may increase breathlessness in clients with COPD. A position that generally helps such clients is sitting upright (high Fowler's position).

4. Schedule respiratory therapy for the afternoon - Incorrect. This does not address the immediate need of the client.

For the NCLEX, understanding the immediate needs and prioritization of care for patients with impaired ventilation/oxygenation is crucial. This can mean knowing how to implement non-pharmacological interventions, proper positioning, medication administration, and coordinating with other healthcare professionals. Always remember, patient safety and immediate needs take priority.

Question 101

A nurse is evaluating the effectiveness of a treatment plan for a client with heart failure who has been prescribed furosemide (Lasix) to manage fluid overload. Which of the following client findings would indicate the treatment plan is effective?

1. The client reports increased shortness of breath.
2. The client's weight has increased by 1 kg in the past week.
3. The client's urine output is 1500 mL over an 8-hour shift.
4. The client's heart rate has increased from 75 to 95 bpm.

Answer Key
The correct answer is 3.

Topic: Evaluating Effectiveness of Treatment Plan for Acute or Chronic Diagnosis

Evaluating the effectiveness of a treatment plan is a critical aspect of nursing practice. This process involves assessing the client's response to treatment, monitoring for changes in the client's condition, and adjusting the care plan as needed based on these observations.

Looking at the options:
1. The client reports increased shortness of breath - Incorrect. An increase in shortness of breath could indicate worsening heart failure and fluid overload, which suggests that the treatment plan may not be effective.
2. The client's weight has increased by 1 kg in the past week - Incorrect. Weight gain could suggest fluid retention, indicating that the furosemide may not be managing the fluid overload effectively.
3. The client's urine output is 1500 mL over an 8-hour shift - Correct. Furosemide is a diuretic, and its therapeutic effect involves increasing urine output to reduce fluid overload. Thus, an increase in urine output is an expected and desired outcome that indicates the medication is working effectively.
4. The client's heart rate has increased from 75 to 95 bpm - Incorrect. An increased heart rate could

indicate that the client's body is working harder to pump blood, possibly due to fluid overload. This is not a desired outcome.

For the NCLEX exam, understanding how to evaluate the effectiveness of a treatment plan is crucial. It requires knowledge about the intended outcomes of prescribed medications and treatments, as well as the ability to interpret changes in the client's condition in relation to these intended outcomes. This ensures that any necessary adjustments to the care plan can be made promptly to optimize the client's health status.

Question 102

A nurse is caring for a client who suddenly becomes unresponsive and pulseless while sitting in a chair. Which of the following actions should the nurse take first?

1. Begin chest compressions.
2. Place the client on the floor.
3. Give two rescue breaths.
4. Attach the automated external defibrillator (AED).

Answer Key
The correct answer is 2.

Topic: Performing Emergency Care Procedures

In emergency situations, it's essential for the nurse to know and follow the appropriate steps in order. This follows the American Heart Association's guidelines for Basic Life Support (BLS), which employs the "CAB" mnemonic: Compressions, Airway, Breathing.

Looking at the options:
1. Begin chest compressions - Incorrect. While initiating chest compressions is a crucial step in cardiopulmonary resuscitation (CPR), the first step should be to ensure the client is in a safe and appropriate position for effective chest compressions.
2. Place the client on the floor - Correct. If a client becomes unresponsive and pulseless while in a chair, the nurse should first move the client to the floor. This is important to provide a firm surface for effective chest compressions and also to ensure the safety of the client during the resuscitation attempt.
3. Give two rescue breaths - Incorrect. Before giving rescue breaths, it's important to begin chest compressions immediately and then open the airway to give breaths.
4. Attach the automated external defibrillator (AED) - Incorrect. While using an AED is crucial during a cardiac arrest situation, the first priority is to place the

301

client on a flat, firm surface to perform chest compressions and ventilation.

To prepare for the NCLEX, it's vital to understand and remember the correct sequence for emergency care procedures. Effective, high-quality chest compressions and early defibrillation are the keys to survival in cardiac arrest, but these measures must be taken in the right order. First, ensure the patient's environment is safe for resuscitation, then start chest compressions, open the airway, give breaths, and use an AED as soon as available.

Question 103

A nurse is caring for a client with chronic obstructive pulmonary disease (COPD). Which of the following pathophysiological changes is the nurse most likely to find in this client?

1. Bronchial constriction and increased mucus production.
2. Alveolar rupture and lung hyperinflation.
3. Increased lung compliance and decreased surfactant production.
4. Restricted lung expansion and interstitial fibrosis.

Answer Key
The correct answer is 2.

Topic: Pathophysiology Related to Acute or Chronic Conditions

COPD is a chronic disease that affects the respiratory system. It involves two main conditions: emphysema and chronic bronchitis. The former is characterized by alveolar rupture and lung hyperinflation, and the latter involves bronchial constriction and increased mucus production. While both conditions occur in people with COPD, the most distinctive pathological change that COPD brings is the alveolar rupture and lung hyperinflation, often more related to emphysema.

Let's break down the options:
1. Bronchial constriction and increased mucus production - Incorrect. This is typically associated with chronic bronchitis and asthma, not the most distinctive feature in COPD.
2. Alveolar rupture and lung hyperinflation - Correct. These are the primary pathophysiological changes seen in emphysema, a type of COPD. The destruction of alveoli results in fewer, larger air sacs and less surface area for gas exchange.
3. Increased lung compliance and decreased surfactant production - Incorrect. This is more indicative of a condition like Acute Respiratory Distress Syndrome (ARDS).

4. Restricted lung expansion and interstitial fibrosis - Incorrect. These features are more characteristic of restrictive lung diseases such as idiopathic pulmonary fibrosis.

Understanding pathophysiology is crucial for the NCLEX. The way diseases modify normal body functions allows healthcare professionals to predict their course, anticipate complications, guide treatment, and educate the patient or family. For the NCLEX, this knowledge will aid in decision-making related to patient symptoms, diagnostic testing, and response to treatment, which are all critical components of effective nursing care.

Question 104

A nurse is monitoring a patient who underwent abdominal surgery 48 hours ago. Which of the following signs should prompt the nurse to suspect a possible complication?

1. The patient reports mild discomfort at the surgical site.
2. The patient's wound is clean and dry with slight swelling.
3. The patient's bowel sounds are audible and regular.
4. The patient is feeling shortness of breath.

Answer Key
The correct answer is 4.

Topic: Recognizing Signs and Symptoms of Client Complications

Recognizing signs and symptoms of complications after surgery is critical in nursing care. Early detection allows for prompt intervention and can prevent further deterioration of the client's health status.

1. Mild discomfort at the surgical site - Incorrect. Mild discomfort at the surgical site within the first few days postoperatively is a normal part of the healing process and not typically indicative of a complication.
2. The patient's wound is clean and dry with slight swelling - Incorrect. A clean and dry wound with slight swelling is typical after surgery. Any redness, increased pain, purulent discharge, or foul odor from the wound should be cause for concern.
3. The patient's bowel sounds are audible and regular - Incorrect. Audible and regular bowel sounds are a positive sign, suggesting that the gastrointestinal system is recovering as expected.
4. The patient is experiencing shortness of breath - Correct. These symptoms can indicate a serious complication such as a pulmonary embolism, which is a medical emergency. This condition can occur postoperatively, especially in clients who are immobile or have other risk factors.

For the NCLEX, candidates must be well-versed in recognizing and responding to signs and symptoms of potential complications in their clients. This requires a solid understanding of the normal healing process and potential complications associated with different types of surgeries or medical treatments. The ability to detect abnormal findings promptly allows for quick intervention and improved patient outcomes.

Question 105

A nurse is caring for a client who has a urinary catheter in place and has suddenly developed a fever, chills, and lower back pain. What is the most appropriate nursing intervention?

1. Increase fluid intake to flush out the bacteria from the urinary tract.
2. Arrange for the client to undergo an immediate surgical procedure.
3. Remove the urinary catheter.
4. Administer antipyretics and wait for symptoms to subside.

Answer Key
The correct answer is 1.

Topic: Intervening as Needed for Client Complications

Intervening promptly in the event of client complications is crucial in nursing. The nurse's role involves recognizing early signs and symptoms of complications and taking appropriate action to mitigate the adverse effects.

1. Increase fluid intake to flush out the bacteria from the urinary tract - Correct. The client's symptoms suggest a urinary tract infection (UTI), possibly related to the catheter. Increasing fluid intake can help flush bacteria out of the urinary tract, which may reduce infection and discomfort. This should be combined with other interventions like obtaining a urine sample for culture and sensitivity, and then, based on the result, the physician can prescribe appropriate antibiotics.
2. Arrange for the client to undergo an immediate surgical procedure - Incorrect. These symptoms do not necessitate immediate surgery. The nurse needs to identify the probable cause (e.g., UTI) and manage accordingly.
3. Remove the urinary catheter - Incorrect. The removal of a urinary catheter should only be done on the physician's orders. In the presence of a UTI, the catheter might be replaced to prevent further infection.

4. Administer antipyretics and wait for symptoms to subside - Incorrect. While antipyretics can help control the fever, they will not address the potential UTI causing the symptoms. Further investigation and treatment are necessary.

The NCLEX emphasizes the nurse's ability to intervene effectively in the presence of client complications. This involves critical thinking, sound clinical judgment, and an understanding of the likely causes and appropriate treatments for various symptoms and complications. Having this knowledge can contribute significantly to improving client outcomes.

Question 106

A client is recently diagnosed with congestive heart failure. The nurse understands that teaching about which of the following lifestyle modifications is MOST beneficial for this client?

1. Engaging in high-intensity exercises regularly.
2. Limiting fluid and sodium intake.
3. Adopting a vegetarian diet.
4. Implementing relaxation techniques such as yoga and meditation.

Answer Key

The correct answer is 2.

Topic: Cardiovascular System Disorders

The management of cardiovascular system disorders, such as congestive heart failure (CHF), demands a deep understanding of the disease process and its implications. Lifestyle modification plays a critical role in managing CHF and other cardiovascular diseases.

1. Engaging in high-intensity exercises regularly - Incorrect. This could increase the heart's workload, worsening the symptoms of CHF. Moderate exercise under medical supervision can be beneficial, but it should be individualized based on the client's health status.
2. Limiting fluid and sodium intake - Correct. This helps to control the volume status and reduce the workload of the heart. Sodium retains water in the body, which can worsen fluid overload, a common issue in CHF. Similarly, limiting fluid intake can help manage fluid overload.
3. Adopting a vegetarian diet - Incorrect. While a healthy diet is essential, it doesn't specifically address the needs of a client with CHF. Limiting sodium and fluid intake are the most critical dietary changes needed.
4. Implementing relaxation techniques such as yoga and meditation - Incorrect. While these may help manage stress and promote general well-being, they do not

directly address the physiological issues associated with CHF.

Preparing for the NCLEX involves understanding not only the pathophysiology of disorders but also their management, including lifestyle modifications. For cardiovascular disorders, these might involve dietary changes, medication management, and modifications to physical activity. This knowledge helps in providing holistic care to the client and significantly improves health outcomes.

Question 107

A client with chronic obstructive pulmonary disease (COPD) is experiencing exacerbation of symptoms. Which of the following interventions should the nurse prioritize?

1. Teaching the client to use a metered-dose inhaler.
2. Administering high-flow oxygen.
3. Encouraging the client to consume a high-protein diet.
4. Assisting with ambulation.

Answer Key
The correct answer is 1.

Topic: Respiratory System Disorders

Chronic obstructive pulmonary disease (COPD) is a chronic, progressive lung disease characterized by difficulty breathing, cough, mucus (sputum) production, and wheezing. It's often caused by long-term exposure to irritating gases or particulate matter, most often from cigarette smoke.

1. Teaching the client to use a metered-dose inhaler - Correct. During an exacerbation of COPD, the priority is to improve the client's respiratory status. The use of a bronchodilator via a metered-dose inhaler can help open the airways, allowing the client to breathe more easily.
2. Administering high-flow oxygen - Incorrect. Although oxygen is usually necessary in cases of COPD exacerbation, care should be taken to avoid giving high-flow oxygen. Many clients with COPD are used to low levels of oxygen, and excessive oxygen can suppress their breathing drive.
3. Encouraging the client to consume a high-protein diet - Incorrect. Although a high-protein diet is important for clients with COPD to prevent malnutrition and maintain strength, it is not the priority during an exacerbation.
4. Assisting with ambulation - Incorrect. While activity is important for maintaining overall health, it is not the priority during an exacerbation of COPD.

In the context of the NCLEX, understanding the complexities of managing respiratory system disorders such as COPD is crucial. The nurse must prioritize interventions that immediately address the client's most acute symptoms and stabilize their condition. In this case, ensuring the client can effectively use a metered-dose inhaler to improve breathing is paramount.

Question 108

A client has been diagnosed with osteoarthritis. The nurse understands that this client is at risk for which of the following complications?

1. Bone deformity.
2. Fluid retention.
3. Hypertension.
4. Decreased appetite.

Answer Key
The correct answer is 1.

Topic: Musculoskeletal System Disorders

Osteoarthritis is a degenerative joint disease, also known as "wear and tear" arthritis. It's the most common form of arthritis, and it occurs when the protective cartilage on the ends of your bones wears down over time.

1. Bone deformity - Correct. Osteoarthritis is characterized by the progressive deterioration of the cartilage in the joints, which can lead to bone deformities. As the condition progresses, the bones may rub together, leading to the formation of bone spurs (osteophytes), which can alter the shape and alignment of the bones.
2. Fluid retention - Incorrect. Although inflammation may occur in the affected joints, osteoarthritis does not typically cause systemic fluid retention.
3. Hypertension - Incorrect. Hypertension is not a direct complication of osteoarthritis. While pain and reduced mobility from osteoarthritis can potentially contribute to a less active lifestyle, which could indirectly impact blood pressure, it is not a direct correlation.
4. Decreased appetite - Incorrect. Decreased appetite is not a direct complication of osteoarthritis. Pain and discomfort can potentially impact appetite but it is not a primary concern with this condition.

In the context of the NCLEX, understanding the implications of musculoskeletal disorders like osteoarthritis is crucial. It's important to be aware of the potential complications, including bone deformities and pain, which can greatly impact a client's quality of life. Nursing interventions for these clients may include pain management, promoting physical mobility, and providing education about the disease and its management. Remember, the priority for clients with osteoarthritis is to manage pain, maintain or improve joint function, and minimize disability. This is often achieved through a combination of treatment strategies, including medication, physical activity, weight management, joint protection, self-management education, and surgery, if necessary.

Question 109

A patient has been diagnosed with psoriasis. Which of the following symptoms would the nurse most likely observe?

1. Small, fluid-filled blisters.
2. Red patches of skin covered with thick, silvery scales.
3. Dark, velvety patches in body folds and creases.
4. Slow-healing sores, especially on the feet and legs.

Answer Key
The correct answer is 2.

Topic: Integumentary System Disorders

Psoriasis is a chronic skin condition caused by an overactive immune system. It involves a rapid buildup of skin cells that forms scales and red patches that are often itchy and sometimes painful.

1. Small, fluid-filled blisters - Incorrect. This is more characteristic of conditions like herpes or shingles, not psoriasis.
2. Red patches of skin covered with thick, silvery scales - Correct. This is a classic presentation of psoriasis. The buildup of skin cells creates scales and red patches that can be itchy or painful.
3. Dark, velvety patches in body folds and creases - Incorrect. This description is more indicative of a condition called acanthosis nigricans, which is often associated with insulin resistance.
4. Slow-healing sores, especially on the feet and legs - Incorrect. While psoriasis can affect any area of the body, this description is more aligned with conditions like diabetic ulcers or peripheral vascular disease.

The NCLEX exam will test your understanding of various integumentary system disorders, including psoriasis. It's critical to be able to identify the unique characteristics of different skin disorders to provide appropriate care and education to patients.

In the context of psoriasis, nursing care includes helping patients manage their symptoms, teaching them about their condition, and reinforcing the need for ongoing medical care. Nurses can also provide emotional support to patients, as skin conditions like psoriasis can have a significant psychological impact due to their visibility.

Non-pharmacological interventions can play a crucial role in managing psoriasis. These may include advising patients to avoid trigger factors that can exacerbate the condition, such as stress, certain medications, skin injury, or smoking. In addition, nursing interventions may include teaching about the importance of moisturizing the skin, using prescribed medications correctly, and recognizing signs of infection. Since psoriasis is a chronic condition, patient education and effective communication between the healthcare provider and patient are vital in managing this condition effectively.

Question 110

A nurse is caring for a patient with Crohn's disease. Which of the following symptoms is the nurse most likely to observe?

1. Dysphagia and a feeling of food stuck in the throat.
2. Colicky abdominal pain and bloody diarrhea.
3. Grey, foul-smelling stool.
4. Severe, sharp pain in the upper abdomen and back.

Answer Key
The correct answer is 2.

Topic: Gastrointestinal System Disorders

Crohn's disease is an inflammatory bowel disease (IBD) that causes inflammation of the digestive tract leading to severe diarrhea, abdominal pain, fatigue, weight loss, and malnutrition.

1. Dysphagia and a feeling of food stuck in the throat - Incorrect. These symptoms are more commonly associated with conditions affecting the esophagus, such as esophageal stricture or achalasia, rather than Crohn's disease.
2. Colicky abdominal pain and bloody diarrhea - Correct. These symptoms are typical of Crohn's disease. The disease often affects the lower part of the small intestine, leading to inflammation and these characteristic symptoms.
3. Grey, foul-smelling stool - Incorrect. This description is more indicative of steatorrhea, which results from malabsorption of fats due to conditions such as pancreatitis or cystic fibrosis.
4. Severe, sharp pain in the upper abdomen and back - Incorrect. While abdominal pain can occur in Crohn's disease, this particular description is more typical of acute pancreatitis.

For the NCLEX exam, understanding the various gastrointestinal disorders, including Crohn's disease, is essential. Recognizing the specific signs and symptoms of each condition enables appropriate and timely interventions. Nursing care for patients with Crohn's disease includes symptom management, dietary guidance, promoting rest, stress management, and patient education about the chronic nature of the disease. Medication administration and monitoring are also crucial, as patients may be prescribed anti-inflammatory drugs, immune system suppressors, antibiotics, or pain relievers.

Patients may need guidance regarding dietary choices, as certain foods can exacerbate symptoms. For instance, spicy foods, high-fiber foods, and dairy products may worsen symptoms for some individuals. A dietitian's consultation may be helpful in these cases.

Additionally, the nurse can provide emotional support, as the chronic nature of Crohn's disease and its impact on quality of life can lead to psychological issues like depression or anxiety. It's also essential for nurses to coordinate with the healthcare team to ensure comprehensive care for these patients.

Question 111

A nurse is caring for a patient with Addison's disease. Which of the following symptoms would most likely be observed?

1. Rapid weight gain and buffalo hump.
2. Irritability and mood changes.
3. Low blood pressure and fatigue.
4. Increased urination and extreme thirst.

Answer Key
The correct answer is 3.

Topic: Endocrine System Disorders

Addison's disease, also known as primary adrenal insufficiency, occurs when the adrenal glands do not produce enough cortisol and, sometimes, aldosterone. This can lead to a range of symptoms and can be life-threatening.

1. Rapid weight gain and buffalo hump - Incorrect. These symptoms are more typically associated with Cushing's syndrome, a condition characterized by excessive cortisol production, not Addison's disease.
2. Irritability and mood changes - Incorrect. While these can be symptoms of various endocrine disorders, they are not the most common or specific signs of Addison's disease.
3. Low blood pressure and fatigue - Correct. Addison's disease can result in low blood pressure (hypotension), due to inadequate aldosterone, and chronic fatigue, due to insufficient cortisol.
4. Increased urination and extreme thirst - Incorrect. These are classic symptoms of diabetes mellitus, specifically indicative of hyperglycemia, not Addison's disease.

For the NCLEX exam, understanding different endocrine disorders, such as Addison's disease, is crucial. Recognizing characteristic signs and symptoms allows for appropriate and timely interventions.

Nursing care for patients with Addison's disease involves administering prescribed medications (usually glucocorticoids and mineralocorticoids), monitoring vital signs (particularly blood pressure), and assessing for signs of Addisonian crisis, a life-threatening condition that can cause severe abdominal pain, low blood pressure, and loss of consciousness.

Patient education is another important nursing role. Patients with Addison's disease need to understand the importance of taking their medications regularly and exactly as prescribed. They should also be instructed to wear a medical alert bracelet and to have extra medication on hand in case of emergencies, as stress can exacerbate symptoms.

It's also critical for nurses to understand the potential complications of Addison's disease, such as Addisonian crisis, and to know how to intervene appropriately. Collaboration with the healthcare team, including the endocrinologist, is vital to ensure comprehensive care for these patients.

Question 112

A nurse is caring for a client diagnosed with chronic kidney disease (CKD). The client's lab reports reveal a decreased glomerular filtration rate (GFR) and elevated serum creatinine. Which nursing intervention would be most appropriate?

1. Encouraging high protein diet
2. Assisting with ambulation four times a day
3. Educating the client about the importance of dialysis
4. Discouraging fluid intake

Answer Key
The correct answer is 3.

Topic: Genitourinary System Disorders

Chronic kidney disease (CKD) is a gradual loss of kidney function over time. Two key markers of kidney function are the glomerular filtration rate (GFR) and serum creatinine levels. In CKD, the GFR decreases, indicating reduced kidney function, and serum creatinine increases as the kidneys lose their ability to filter this waste product.

1. Encouraging a high protein diet - Incorrect. A diet high in protein can put more strain on the kidneys, leading to an accumulation of waste products in the blood, which the impaired kidneys cannot efficiently eliminate. A low to moderate protein diet is often recommended in CKD.
2. Assisting with ambulation four times a day - Incorrect. While physical activity is important for overall health, this intervention is not directly related to managing CKD or its symptoms.
3. Educating the client about the importance of dialysis - Correct. Dialysis can replace some of the kidneys' function by removing waste products from the blood. Education about dialysis, its importance, and how it works is crucial in CKD management, especially when the disease progresses to the point where dialysis may be needed.
4. Discouraging fluid intake - Incorrect. Fluid intake in CKD needs to be individualized, depending on the

patient's urine output and presence of edema or hypertension. Therefore, discouraging fluid intake is not necessarily appropriate without further information.

As a nurse preparing for the NCLEX, understanding the pathophysiology, clinical manifestations, and nursing management of genitourinary disorders such as CKD is vital. Key nursing interventions for CKD include monitoring vital signs, providing patient education about the disease and its management, monitoring lab results (e.g., GFR, serum creatinine, electrolytes), managing symptoms (e.g., fatigue, anemia, pruritus), and supporting the patient emotionally.

Additionally, it's crucial to work closely with the healthcare team, including nephrologists and dietitians, to provide comprehensive care. For example, dietitians can provide valuable guidance on dietary modifications that can help manage CKD, such as limiting protein, sodium, potassium, and phosphorus intake. Always remember, the ultimate goal is to slow the progression of the disease, manage symptoms, and prevent complications.

Question 113

A nurse is providing care to a client who has just been diagnosed with Systemic Lupus Erythematosus (SLE). Which of the following statements by the client indicates a need for further teaching?

1. "I should avoid going out in the sun without protection."
2. "I need to report any signs of a fever or sore throat to my doctor."
3. "I should expect to have regular blood tests."
4. "I can stop taking my medication when my symptoms go away."

Answer Key
The correct answer is 4.

Topic: Immune System Disorders

Systemic Lupus Erythematosus (SLE), also known as lupus, is a chronic autoimmune disease characterized by inflammation and damage to various body tissues. It's a complex disorder that can affect the skin, joints, kidneys, brain, and other organs.

1. "I should avoid going out in the sun without protection." - This is a correct understanding. Sun exposure can trigger lupus flares, so sun protection is vital.
2. "I need to report any signs of a fever or sore throat to my doctor." - This is a correct understanding. A fever or sore throat could indicate an infection, which can exacerbate lupus or be a sign of lupus flare.
3. "I should expect to have regular blood tests." - This is a correct understanding. Regular blood tests monitor the disease's progression and the effect of medication.
4. "I can stop taking my medication when my symptoms go away." - This statement indicates a need for further teaching. It's crucial to continue taking medication as prescribed, even when symptoms improve, to control the disease and prevent flares.

In preparing for the NCLEX, understand the pathophysiology, clinical manifestations, and nursing interventions for immune disorders like SLE. Remember that SLE's symptoms can vary greatly from person to person. Common symptoms include fatigue, joint pain and swelling, skin rashes, and fever. More severe symptoms may involve the kidneys, heart, lungs, or other organs.

Nursing interventions often involve patient education on medication adherence, lifestyle modifications (such as sun protection and a balanced diet), regular healthcare visits, and symptom monitoring. It's also essential to address psychosocial aspects of care, as living with a chronic illness like SLE can be challenging and may lead to stress, anxiety, or depression.

Lastly, coordinating care with a multidisciplinary team, including physicians, physical therapists, social workers, and dietitians, can help provide comprehensive care to clients with SLE.

Question 114

A nurse is caring for a patient with Parkinson's disease. Which of the following symptoms is a key feature of this neurological disorder?

1. Memory loss and disorientation.
2. Tremors at rest and bradykinesia.
3. Severe muscle spasms and hypertonicity.
4. Involuntary eye movements and difficulty walking.

Answer Key
The correct answer is 2.

Topic: Nervous System Disorders

Parkinson's disease (PD) is a neurodegenerative disorder affecting the dopaminergic neurons in the substantia nigra area of the brain. This area is responsible for coordinating movement, so Parkinson's disease primarily results in motor symptoms. However, non-motor symptoms also occur and can significantly impact the person's quality of life.

1. "Memory loss and disorientation" - While cognitive changes can occur in Parkinson's disease, particularly in the later stages, they are not a key feature. These symptoms are more characteristic of dementia such as Alzheimer's disease.
2. "Tremors at rest and bradykinesia" - This is the correct choice. A classic feature of Parkinson's disease is rest tremor, which usually starts in one hand and then may progress to affect other body parts. Bradykinesia, or slowness of movement, is another common feature of Parkinson's disease.
3. "Severe muscle spasms and hypertonicity" - These symptoms are more characteristic of conditions like spastic cerebral palsy or multiple sclerosis, not Parkinson's disease.
4. "Involuntary eye movements and difficulty walking" - Involuntary eye movements are more characteristic of conditions like nystagmus, not Parkinson's disease. Although difficulty walking can occur in Parkinson's

due to bradykinesia and postural instability, it is not paired with involuntary eye movements.

The management of Parkinson's disease includes medication therapy (e.g., Levodopa-Carbidopa), surgery in some cases (like deep brain stimulation), and comprehensive care involving physical, occupational, and speech therapy. Nurses play a crucial role in patient education, medication management, safety promotion, and coordination of care among the healthcare team. Understanding the pathophysiology, symptomatology, and management strategies for Parkinson's disease is critical for the NCLEX examination.

Question 115

A nurse is caring for a patient who has been recently diagnosed with polycythemia vera. Which of the following signs and symptoms would the nurse expect to observe?

1. Shortness of breath and fatigue.
2. Frequent nosebleeds and bruising.
3. Itching and ruddy complexion.
4. Weight loss and night sweats.

Answer Key
The correct answer is 3.

Topic: Hematological Disorders

Polycythemia vera is a type of blood disorder that results in an overproduction of red blood cells. This leads to thicker blood, which can cause a host of symptoms and increase the risk of developing blood clots.

1. "Shortness of breath and fatigue" - These symptoms are more characteristic of anemia, a condition marked by a lack of healthy red blood cells or hemoglobin, not polycythemia vera.
2. "Frequent nosebleeds and bruising" - While these symptoms can occur in various blood disorders, they are not specific to polycythemia vera and are often more associated with clotting disorders.
3. "Itching and ruddy complexion" - This is the correct choice. Itching, especially after a hot shower, and a ruddy (red) complexion, particularly in the face, are common symptoms of polycythemia vera due to the overproduction of red blood cells.
4. "Weight loss and night sweats" - These symptoms are often associated with lymphomas and other types of cancers, not specifically with polycythemia vera.

The management of polycythemia vera aims to reduce the blood's thickness, manage symptoms, and prevent complications, such as blood clots. This is usually achieved through phlebotomy (removal of blood from the body), medication, and aspirin. Nurses play a key role in managing the symptoms, educating patients about the disease and treatment, and monitoring for potential complications. As a candidate preparing for the NCLEX exam, you should understand the common signs, symptoms, and treatment approaches for various hematological disorders, including polycythemia vera.

Question 116

A nurse is providing discharge education to a patient who has been diagnosed with age-related macular degeneration (AMD). Which of the following statements made by the patient indicates a need for further teaching?

1. "I understand that my central vision will be most affected by this condition."
2. "I can slow the progression of AMD by quitting smoking and eating a diet rich in fruits and vegetables."
3. "Regular eye examinations will not help because AMD is not treatable."
4. "I should monitor my vision regularly using an Amsler grid."

Answer Key

The correct answer is 3.

Topic: Eye Disorders

Age-related macular degeneration (AMD) is a leading cause of vision loss among people aged 50 and older. It causes damage to the macula, a small spot near the center of the retina, which is required for sharp, clear central vision.

1. "I understand that my central vision will be most affected by this condition." - This statement is correct. AMD affects central vision, leading to difficulty in activities requiring sharp vision such as reading and driving.
2. "I can slow the progression of AMD by quitting smoking and eating a diet rich in fruits and vegetables." - This statement is accurate. Lifestyle modifications like quitting smoking and consuming a balanced diet rich in antioxidants can help slow the progression of AMD.
3. "Regular eye examinations will not help because AMD is not treatable." - This statement is incorrect, hence the need for further teaching. While there's no cure for AMD, regular eye examinations can help detect the condition early and manage its progression with treatments like anti-VEGF drugs, laser therapy, and photodynamic therapy.
4. "I should monitor my vision regularly using an Amsler grid." - This statement is correct. An Amsler grid is a

tool that can help patients with AMD monitor their vision and notice any changes or distortions.

For the NCLEX exam, you should be familiar with common eye disorders, their symptoms, management strategies, and important patient teaching points. Understanding the impact of lifestyle factors on disease progression and the importance of regular monitoring in conditions like AMD is also crucial.

Question 117

A nurse is caring for a patient recently diagnosed with Ménière's disease. Which of the following statements, if made by the patient, would indicate a need for further teaching?

1. "I may experience episodes of vertigo due to my condition."
2. "My hearing loss is temporary and will improve after a few weeks."
3. "A low-salt diet can help manage my symptoms."
4. "I should avoid sudden movements to decrease my symptoms."

Answer Key
The correct answer is 2.

Topic: Ear Disorders

Ménière's disease is an inner ear disorder that can cause a variety of symptoms such as vertigo, tinnitus (ringing in the ear), hearing loss, and a feeling of fullness in the ear. The condition is chronic and usually affects only one ear.

1. "I may experience episodes of vertigo due to my condition." - This statement is accurate. Ménière's disease can cause severe dizziness (vertigo), often accompanied by nausea and vomiting.
2. "My hearing loss is temporary and will improve after a few weeks." - This statement is incorrect, which indicates the need for further teaching. Hearing loss in Ménière's disease is usually progressive and can be permanent.
3. "A low-salt diet can help manage my symptoms." - This statement is true. A diet low in sodium can help reduce fluid buildup in the inner ear, thereby reducing the severity and frequency of Ménière's disease symptoms.
4. "I should avoid sudden movements to decrease my symptoms." - This statement is correct. Sudden movements or position changes can trigger vertigo attacks in individuals with Ménière's disease.

For the NCLEX exam, understanding various ear disorders, their symptoms, and management is crucial. You should be familiar with patient education points, including dietary modifications and lifestyle changes that can help manage these conditions.

Question 118

A nurse is caring for a client who has been diagnosed with oral candidiasis. Which of the following patient statements indicates understanding of the condition and its treatment?

1. "I should rinse my mouth with water after using my prescribed antifungal mouthwash."
2. "I'll eat more spicy foods to help kill the fungus."
3. "It's okay for me to share my toothbrush with my spouse."
4. "I will stop my treatment once my symptoms have disappeared."

Answer Key
The correct answer is 1.

Topic: Nose, Mouth, and Throat Disorders

Oral candidiasis, also known as oral thrush, is a condition caused by the overgrowth of a type of yeast called Candida in the mouth. It can cause symptoms like creamy white lesions on the tongue or inner cheeks, mouth pain, and difficulty swallowing.

1. "I should rinse my mouth with water after using my prescribed antifungal mouthwash." - This statement is correct. The client should not rinse their mouth with water immediately after using an antifungal mouthwash as it can wash away the medicine.
2. "I'll eat more spicy foods to help kill the fungus." - This statement is incorrect. There's no evidence to suggest that spicy foods can help to kill Candida.
3. "It's okay for me to share my toothbrush with my spouse." - This statement is incorrect. Sharing personal items like toothbrushes can spread the Candida fungus.
4. "I will stop my treatment once my symptoms have disappeared." - This statement is incorrect. Treatment should be continued for the full course, even if symptoms disappear before then, to ensure the infection is fully treated and to reduce the risk of recurrence.

For the NCLEX exam, understanding the different types of disorders affecting the nose, mouth, and throat, and their treatment protocols is important. Candidates should be aware of patient education points for these conditions, including treatment adherence, maintaining oral hygiene, and avoiding sharing personal items like toothbrushes.

Question 119

A male client has been diagnosed with benign prostatic hyperplasia (BPH). Which of the following statements by the client indicates a correct understanding of his condition?

1. "I will need to have my prostate completely removed."
2. "I might experience erectile dysfunction as a result of this condition."
3. "This condition increases my risk for developing prostate cancer."
4. "I can expect frequent, urgent needs to urinate."

Answer Key
The correct answer is 4.

Topic: Reproductive System Disorders

Benign prostatic hyperplasia (BPH) is a common condition in older men where the prostate gland enlarges and can cause problems with urination. The exact cause is unknown, but it's believed to be related to changes in sex hormones as a man ages.

1. "I will need to have my prostate completely removed." - This statement is incorrect. While surgery is a possible treatment option for BPH, it's not usually the first line of treatment and doesn't necessarily involve removing the entire prostate.
2. "I might experience erectile dysfunction as a result of this condition." - This statement is incorrect. BPH does not cause erectile dysfunction. However, some treatments for BPH can have side effects that could affect sexual function.
3. "This condition increases my risk for developing prostate cancer." - This statement is incorrect. Despite both conditions involving the prostate, there is no scientific evidence that BPH increases the risk of prostate cancer.
4. "I can expect frequent, urgent needs to urinate." - This statement is correct. BPH can cause urination problems, including increased frequency and urgency of urination, especially at night (nocturia).

For the NCLEX exam, it's important to understand the various reproductive system disorders, their causes, symptoms, and treatment options. Education and communication with clients about their conditions and what to expect can significantly contribute to their understanding and management of their condition. This promotes better health outcomes and improves their quality of life.

Question 120

A pregnant woman in her third trimester comes to the clinic with complaints of visual disturbances, headache, and swelling of her hands and face. Based on these symptoms, the nurse should suspect which of the following conditions?

1. Preeclampsia
2. Gestational diabetes
3. Placenta previa
4. Hyperemesis gravidarum

Answer Key
The correct answer is 1.

Topic: Pregnancy and Childbirth Related Disorders

Preeclampsia is a pregnancy complication characterized by high blood pressure and signs of damage to another organ system, often the liver and kidneys. This condition usually begins after 20 weeks of pregnancy in women whose blood pressure had been normal.

1. "Preeclampsia" - This is the correct answer. The symptoms mentioned are classic signs of preeclampsia, which includes high blood pressure, swelling (edema), sudden weight gain from retaining fluids, and protein in the urine. Other signs and symptoms may include severe headaches, changes in vision including temporary loss of vision, blurred vision or light sensitivity, upper abdominal pain, nausea or vomiting, decreased urine output, and shortness of breath.
2. "Gestational diabetes" - While gestational diabetes can cause complications in pregnancy, the symptoms presented do not align with this condition. Gestational diabetes is primarily diagnosed through an oral glucose tolerance test.
3. "Placenta previa" - This condition is characterized by the placenta partially or fully blocking the cervix, which can lead to bleeding during pregnancy and problems during childbirth. It does not typically present with the symptoms described.

4. "Hyperemesis gravidarum" - This is a severe form of morning sickness that leads to weight loss and dehydration, not the symptoms listed in the question.

For the NCLEX exam, understanding the common complications related to pregnancy and childbirth, their symptoms, management, and nursing care is essential. Nurses play a vital role in identifying these conditions early, providing appropriate care, and preventing further complications.

Question 121

A 1-week-old newborn is brought to the pediatrician's office with a persistent yellowing of the skin and sclera. The nurse should suspect which of the following conditions?

1. Newborn sepsis
2. Neonatal jaundice
3. Newborn cystic fibrosis
4. Neonatal hypoglycemia

Answer Key
The correct answer is 2.

Topic: Newborn and Infant Disorders

Neonatal jaundice is a common condition in newborns due to an excess of bilirubin, a yellow pigment of red blood cells.

1. "Newborn sepsis" - While newborn sepsis is a severe condition requiring immediate intervention, it typically presents with symptoms like fever, lethargy, poor feeding, or respiratory distress. Jaundice can be a symptom, but it's not the most common or definitive one.
2. "Neonatal jaundice" - This is the correct answer. It's characterized by yellowing of a baby's skin and the whites of the eyes. The yellow color is due to an excess amount of bilirubin, a byproduct of the normal breakdown of old red blood cells. Jaundice in newborns usually appears between the second and third days of life.
3. "Newborn cystic fibrosis" - Cystic fibrosis is a serious genetic condition that causes severe damage to the lungs, digestive system, and other organs. It does not typically present as jaundice.
4. "Neonatal hypoglycemia" - While hypoglycemia (low blood sugar) can occur in newborns, the typical symptoms are jitteriness, poor feeding, hypothermia, and lethargy, not jaundice.

For the NCLEX, knowing the common conditions in newborns and infants, how to identify them, and what steps to take for intervention is crucial. Early identification and management can significantly impact the infant's health and development. As a nurse, you're often the first line of defense in noticing changes in a newborn's condition.

Question 122

A 6-year-old boy is brought to the pediatrician's office by his parents, who report that he has had a persistent cough and low-grade fever for the past week. On physical examination, the nurse observes clubbing of the fingers. This symptom is most commonly associated with which of the following conditions?

1. Asthma
2. Cystic fibrosis
3. Allergic rhinitis
4. Pneumonia

Answer Key

The correct answer is 2.

Topic: Pediatric Disorders

Clubbing of the fingers, where the tips of the fingers enlarge and the nails curve around the fingertips, is often associated with conditions that result in chronically low levels of oxygen in the blood, such as cystic fibrosis.

1. "Asthma" - While asthma can cause chronic respiratory symptoms, it is not typically associated with clubbing of the fingers. Symptoms more commonly associated with asthma include shortness of breath, wheezing, and coughing.
2. "Cystic fibrosis" - This is the correct answer. Cystic fibrosis is a genetic disorder that affects the lungs and digestive system, causing severe damage. In cystic fibrosis, a thick, sticky mucus can clog the lungs, leading to life-threatening lung infections. The body's decreased ability to effectively move oxygen into the bloodstream can result in clubbing.
3. "Allergic rhinitis" - This condition is characterized by an allergic response causing itchy, watery eyes, sneezing, and other similar symptoms. It is not associated with clubbing.
4. "Pneumonia" - While pneumonia can result in a cough and low-grade fever, it is an acute infection, and clubbing of the fingers is a sign of chronic oxygen deprivation.

On the NCLEX, it's important to remember that pediatric clients can present differently than adults. Understanding how different diseases can present in this population will be vital in answering questions correctly and providing the best care possible.

Question 123

An 80-year-old client presents with increased confusion and unsteady gait over the past week. The nurse also notes that the client has a new-onset incontinence. Which of the following should the nurse suspect?

1. Alzheimer's disease
2. Urinary tract infection
3. Parkinson's disease
4. Normal aging process

Answer Key
The correct answer is 2.

Topic: Elderly Client Disorders

New onset confusion, unsteady gait, and incontinence in an elderly patient can often indicate an infection, such as a urinary tract infection (UTI). Elderly patients may not exhibit the classic symptoms of UTI like dysuria or fever, instead, they may exhibit altered mental status, falls, incontinence, or even increased agitation.

1. "Alzheimer's disease" - While confusion can occur in Alzheimer's disease, this condition typically presents with a slow, progressive decline in memory and cognitive function, rather than a sudden change over a week.
2. "Urinary tract infection" - This is the correct answer. In older adults, UTIs may cause sudden changes in behavior such as confusion or agitation, unsteady gait, and incontinence. These symptoms are sometimes mistaken for the early signs of dementia or Alzheimer's disease.
3. "Parkinson's disease" - Parkinson's disease can cause gait problems and cognitive changes, but these are typically progressive and would not suddenly appear over the course of a week.
4. "Normal aging process" - While some cognitive changes and unsteadiness can be part of the normal

aging process, sudden onset over a week is not typical and warrants further investigation.

For the NCLEX, it is important to understand that the presentation of common illnesses like UTI can be different in the elderly population. Rather than the common symptoms of fever, pain or burning during urination that are typically seen in younger adults, older adults might present with nonspecific symptoms like confusion, incontinence, or changes in functional status. Always consider UTI when there is a sudden change in behavior or functional status in an elderly patient.

Question 124

A nurse is caring for a client who just underwent surgery and is in severe pain. The physician has ordered morphine 10 mg IV every 4 hours PRN. The client reports that the pain medication is not effective and they are still in severe pain even after the administration of the drug. Which of the following is the most appropriate next step for the nurse?

1. Administer an additional dose of morphine without the doctor's order.
2. Tell the client that nothing more can be done about the pain.
3. Consult with the doctor about the ineffectiveness of the pain medication.
4. Suggest the client distract themselves to help manage the pain.

Answer Key
The correct answer is 3.

Topic: Pharmacological Pain Management

Pain management is a critical aspect of patient care, especially post-surgery. The goal is to ensure that the client is as comfortable as possible, which aids in recovery. Morphine is a strong opioid analgesic often used in severe pain management, such as post-surgery.

1. "Administer an additional dose of morphine without the doctor's order" - This is inappropriate and dangerous. Nurses must always follow the prescribed orders, and not administering additional doses without physician's order as it could lead to overdose or other serious complications.
2. "Tell the client that nothing more can be done about the pain" - This is not therapeutic or accurate. There are always different approaches and medications that can be tried if one is not effective.
3. "Consult with the doctor about the ineffectiveness of the pain medication" - This is the correct answer. If a medication is not effectively managing a client's pain, it is the responsibility of the nurse to advocate for the client and consult with the physician for a possible medication change or adjustment.
4. "Suggest the client distract themselves to help manage the pain" - While distraction can be a useful adjuvant in pain management, it should not be the primary method, especially when dealing with severe

pain. This option could be considered disrespectful and dismissive to the patient's pain.

For the NCLEX, understanding the principles of pain management is key. Always evaluate the effectiveness of pain medications and advocate for your client if pain management is not sufficient. Never administer more medication than ordered by the physician, and do not dismiss a client's pain. Use a pain scale to accurately assess the pain level.

Question 125

A nurse is caring for a client with chronic back pain. The client is interested in trying non-pharmacological methods to manage their pain. Which of the following interventions should the nurse suggest?

1. Increasing the dosage of current pain medications.
2. Guided imagery and deep breathing exercises.
3. Ignoring the pain until it becomes severe.
4. Advising the client to remain in bed and avoid physical activities.

Answer Key
The correct answer is 2.

Topic: Non-Pharmacological Pain Management

Non-pharmacological pain management involves the use of methods other than medication to control pain. These techniques can often be used in conjunction with medication to provide more comprehensive pain relief. Some commonly used non-pharmacological methods for pain management include:

1. Physical methods, such as massage, heat or cold therapy, transcutaneous electrical nerve stimulation (TENS), acupuncture, and physical therapy.
2. Psychological methods, such as relaxation techniques (guided imagery, deep breathing exercises, progressive muscle relaxation), cognitive behavioral therapy, and distraction.
3. Lifestyle changes, including regular exercise, a balanced diet, and maintaining a healthy weight.
4. Let's evaluate each of the options provided:
5. "Increasing the dosage of current pain medications" - This is not a non-pharmacological method and should be done only on a physician's order.
6. "Guided imagery and deep breathing exercises" - This is the correct answer. These are effective non-pharmacological techniques that the client can use to help manage their chronic back pain.
7. "Ignoring the pain until it becomes severe" - This is not an effective or safe strategy for managing pain.

8. "Advising the client to remain in bed and avoid physical activities" - While rest can sometimes be beneficial, long-term bed rest is generally not recommended as it can lead to other complications, such as muscle weakness and atrophy. Physical activity is typically encouraged as part of a comprehensive pain management plan.

Understanding non-pharmacological pain management methods is essential for the NCLEX exam as well as for your nursing practice. These methods can often provide effective pain relief and improve the quality of life for clients dealing with chronic pain.

Question 126

A nurse is providing education to a client with a newly diagnosed atrial fibrillation who has been prescribed warfarin. The client also takes ibuprofen for osteoarthritis pain. Which of the following statements should the nurse include in the teaching?

1. "You can continue taking ibuprofen as you normally do."
2. "Warfarin and ibuprofen do not interact with each other."
3. "Taking warfarin and ibuprofen together can increase your risk of bleeding."
4. "Warfarin will make your ibuprofen less effective."

Answer Key
The correct answer is 3.

Topic: Common Drug Interactions

Drug interactions occur when the effects of one drug are altered by the concurrent administration of another drug (prescription or over-the-counter), food, or even beverages. These interactions can increase or decrease the effectiveness of the drugs or cause unexpected side effects.

In this case, the interaction is between warfarin and ibuprofen. Warfarin is an anticoagulant medication that is commonly used to treat or prevent blood clots. Ibuprofen is a nonsteroidal anti-inflammatory drug (NSAID) often used to treat pain or inflammation.

Both of these medications can increase the risk of bleeding. Warfarin works by decreasing the clotting ability of the blood, while ibuprofen can inhibit platelet aggregation and also cause gastrointestinal bleeding. Therefore, taking these medications together can significantly increase the risk of serious bleeding complications.

As a future nurse preparing for the NCLEX, understanding drug interactions is crucial. It's important to always check for potential drug interactions before administering medications and educate patients about the potential risks of mixing medications. Effective patient education can significantly reduce the risk of harmful drug interactions.

Question 127

A nurse is providing education to a client who has just been started on a course of prednisone for their rheumatoid arthritis. Which of the following information should the nurse include in their teaching?

1. "You may stop taking this medication as soon as your symptoms improve."
2. "You might experience increased appetite and weight gain."
3. "You don't have to worry about any side effects with this medication."
4. "This medication will cure your rheumatoid arthritis."

Answer Key
The correct answer is 2.

Topic: Client Education on Drug Side Effects and Adherence

Patient education regarding medication adherence and side effects is a fundamental part of nursing practice and critical for the NCLEX. Nurses have an important role in ensuring patients understand how to take their medication correctly and what potential side effects may occur.

Prednisone is a corticosteroid medication that is often used to treat inflammatory conditions such as rheumatoid arthritis. While it can be effective at reducing inflammation and pain, it can also cause a number of side effects. One common side effect of prednisone is an increase in appetite, which can lead to weight gain. Other side effects can include mood changes, trouble sleeping, and increased blood sugar levels.

It's also crucial to advise the patient that they should not stop taking this medication abruptly, even if their symptoms improve. Prednisone needs to be tapered under the supervision of a healthcare provider to avoid withdrawal symptoms.

Furthermore, it's essential to clarify to the patient that while prednisone can help manage the symptoms of rheumatoid arthritis, it does not cure the disease. Effective patient education promotes adherence to medication regimens, improves treatment outcomes, and reduces the risk of complications or adverse effects.

Question 128

A nurse is preparing to administer a new medication to a client. Which of the following actions by the nurse would be the best way to assess the client's understanding of the drug therapy?

1. The nurse asks the client to explain what the medication is for.
2. The nurse asks the client if they are allergic to any medications.
3. The nurse reads the medication information leaflet to the client.
4. The nurse asks the client if they have any questions about the medication.

Answer Key
The correct answer is 1.

Topic: Assessing Client Understanding of Drug Therapy

As an NCLEX candidate, it's crucial to understand the importance of assessing a client's understanding of their drug therapy. One effective method is using the "teach-back" method, where the nurse asks the client to explain in their own words what they understand about the medication. This allows the nurse to gauge the client's comprehension and correct any misconceptions right away.

While asking the client if they have any questions about the medication (option 4) is important, it doesn't necessarily assess the client's understanding. The client might not know what questions to ask.

Asking about allergies (option 2) is an essential part of medication safety, but it doesn't measure the client's understanding of the drug therapy.

Reading the medication information leaflet to the client (option 3) is helpful, but it does not evaluate the client's comprehension.

Ensuring the client understands the purpose of the medication, how to take it, possible side effects, and what to do if a dose is missed, among other things, is a critical aspect of patient education and promotes medication adherence and safety. Always remember that patient teaching and assessment of understanding is an ongoing process and should be done each time a new medication is started or when the regimen is changed.

Question 129

A nurse is preparing to administer medications to a client. Which of the following actions is NOT a standard precaution for preventing medication errors?

1. Double-checking all medications against the original order before administration.
2. Administering a medication that another nurse has drawn up or prepared.
3. Using at least two client identifiers before administering medications.
4. Documenting the administration of medication immediately after administration.

Answer Key
The correct answer is 2.

Topic: Medication Error Prevention

For the NCLEX, it's important to remember that safe medication administration is one of the fundamental responsibilities of a nurse. Medication errors can cause significant harm to patients, so adhering to standard precautions is crucial.

Option 2 is the incorrect practice. Nurses should never administer a medication that another nurse has drawn up or prepared. This is because the nurse administering the medication is responsible for ensuring its correctness. If another nurse prepares the medication, there could be a potential for error that the administering nurse could miss.

Option 1 is a key step in medication administration. It's essential to double-check all medications against the original order before administration. This helps to confirm the correct medication, dose, route, and timing.

Option 3 relates to patient identification. The nurse should use at least two client identifiers (such as name and date of birth) before administering medications to ensure the right medication is given to the right patient.

Option 4 is about documentation, which should be done immediately after administration. This is to prevent errors in documentation, such as forgetting to document or documenting the wrong medication or dose.

In the broader context of medication safety, nurses should also be aware of "high-alert" medications, participate in medication reconciliation, and promote a culture of safety where errors can be reported without fear of blame. Ongoing education about medication safety is also vital for maintaining nursing competence and improving patient outcomes.

Question 130

A nurse is performing medication reconciliation for a client recently admitted to the hospital. Which of the following actions should the nurse take FIRST?

1. Check the client's medical records for any documented drug allergies.
2. Call the client's primary care physician to verify their current medications.
3. Ask the client to list all the medications they are currently taking, including over-the-counter (OTC) medications and supplements.
4. Compare the client's list of medications with the medications ordered by the admitting physician.

Answer Key
The correct answer is 3.

Topic: Medication Reconciliation

Medication reconciliation is a key patient safety practice that seeks to prevent adverse drug events by ensuring accurate and complete medication information transfer at interfaces of care.

For the NCLEX, it's important to understand the steps involved in medication reconciliation. The first step is always obtaining the most accurate list possible of all medications the patient is currently taking. This includes not just prescription medications, but also over-the-counter drugs, herbal supplements, vitamins, and any other substances the patient may be taking. This is done by a comprehensive interview with the patient and/or their caregivers. Hence, option 3 is the correct answer.

Option 1, checking the client's medical records for any documented drug allergies, is indeed an important part of medication reconciliation, but it's not the first step. It's part of the verification process which comes after obtaining the medication list from the patient.

Option 2, calling the client's primary care physician to verify their current medications, is also part of the verification process. This is typically done if there are discrepancies or uncertainties after comparing the patient's list with the doctor's orders.

Option 4, comparing the client's list of medications with the medications ordered by the admitting physician, is the next step after collecting the patient's medication list. This process is called "clarification". Any discrepancies identified should be resolved, and all changes, omissions, and discrepancies should be documented and communicated to the patient, caregiver, and appropriate healthcare providers.

Effective medication reconciliation requires strong communication skills, a meticulous approach, and a thorough understanding of medications. Always remember, the goal is to ensure that the patient receives the correct medications at all transitions of care.

Question 131

A nurse is preparing to administer a parenteral medication via intramuscular (IM) route. Which of the following actions should the nurse take?

1. Select a needle gauge between 18 and 25 depending on the viscosity of the medication.
2. Insert the needle at a 90-degree angle into the muscle.
3. Aspirate for a few seconds before administering the medication.
4. Massage the injection site after administering the medication.

Answer Key
The correct answer is 2.

Topic: Administration of Parenteral Medications

Parenteral medication administration is a route of administration that bypasses the digestive tract and involves injecting or infusing medications into the body via routes such as intramuscular (IM), subcutaneous (SubQ), and intravenous (IV).

Intramuscular injections are given when the medication is to be absorbed quickly. For the NCLEX, it's essential to know that when giving an IM injection, the needle should be inserted at a 90-degree angle into the muscle (option 2), making it the correct answer.

Option 1 is partially correct. While it's true that the needle gauge is selected based on the viscosity of the medication, for IM injections, usually a 20-25 gauge needle is used.

Option 3 is no longer a recommended practice for all IM injections. Aspiration was previously taught to ensure that the needle is not in a blood vessel before injecting the medication. However, current guidelines from the Centers for Disease Control and Prevention (CDC) and World Health Organization (WHO) advise against this practice due to lack of evidence that it benefits the patient or prevents complications.

Option 4 is incorrect. It was once a common practice to massage the injection site after giving an IM injection to help distribute the medication. However, current practice guidelines recommend against massaging the site as it may cause tissue irritation, can lead to discomfort, and may disperse the medication too quickly.

The administration of parenteral medications requires accurate knowledge and precision to ensure patient safety. Always follow your facility's policies and procedures when administering medications. Remember to perform the "five rights" before administration: right patient, right medication, right dose, right route, and right time.

Question 132

A nurse is preparing to administer an enteral medication to a patient with a nasogastric (NG) tube. Which of the following actions should the nurse take?

1. Crush the medication and mix it with a large volume of water.
2. Administer the medication while the patient is in a supine position.
3. Verify the placement of the NG tube before administration.
4. Administer the medication directly from the medication cup into the NG tube.

Answer Key
The correct answer is 3.

Topic: Administration of Enteral Medications

Enteral medications are those given through a tube directly into the gastrointestinal tract. This includes oral medications that are converted for administration via a feeding tube like a nasogastric (NG) or gastrostomy tube. For the NCLEX, understanding the correct steps for administering enteral medications is crucial.

The correct action (option 3) is to verify the placement of the NG tube before administration. Checking tube placement ensures the medication is delivered to the correct location and reduces the risk of aspiration.

Option 1 is not entirely correct. While it's true that most solid oral medications can be crushed and mixed with water before being given through a feeding tube, the volume of water used should be appropriate (usually 15-30 mL) and specific to patient needs and medication properties. Some medications should not be crushed due to their design for time-release or enteric coating, for example. Always check medication guidelines or consult a pharmacist if you're unsure.

Option 2 is incorrect because the patient should not be in a supine position when administering enteral medications, as this increases the risk of aspiration. The patient should be in an upright or Fowler's position during administration and for 30 minutes afterward.

Option 4 is incorrect because medications should not be administered directly from the medication cup into the NG tube. The medication should be administered using a syringe to allow for better control of the medication flow and prevent clogging of the tube.

Remember to follow the steps for safe medication administration, including confirming the patient's identity and the five rights: the right patient, the right medication, the right dose, the right route, and the right time. Lastly, always flush the tube before and after each medication administration to maintain patency and prevent drug-drug interactions within the tube.

Question 133

A nurse is preparing to administer a topical medication to a patient with a severe skin rash. Which of the following actions is appropriate?

1. Apply the medication to the most severe areas of the rash first.
2. Apply the medication with a gloved hand.
3. Rub the medication vigorously into the skin.
4. Apply a thick layer of the medication to ensure effectiveness.

Answer Key
The correct answer is 2.

Topic: Administration of Topical Medications

Topical medications are applied directly to the body surfaces, such as the skin or mucous membranes. They can come in various forms, including creams, ointments, patches, and gels, and are often used for their local effect, although some can have systemic effects.

Option 2 is correct. A nurse should always wear gloves when applying topical medications. This practice not only protects the nurse from potential exposure to the drug and the patient's skin condition but also prevents additional contamination of the patient's skin.

Option 1 is not necessarily correct. The application of topical medications should be based on the prescriber's directions and can vary depending on the medication and the condition being treated.

Option 3 is incorrect. Topical medications should not be rubbed vigorously into the skin. Many conditions treated with topical medications can make the skin more sensitive, and vigorous rubbing can cause further irritation or damage. Instead, the medication should be applied gently and evenly over the area.

Option 4 is also incorrect. Applying a thick layer of medication does not necessarily increase its effectiveness and can sometimes lead to problems such as skin irritation or systemic absorption, particularly if the medication is not intended to be used in large quantities. The amount of medication applied should follow the prescriber's instructions.

For the NCLEX, remember the principles of safe medication administration also apply to topical medications. This includes verifying the patient's identity, checking for any allergies, and confirming the right medication, right dose, right route, right time, and right reason before administration. Additionally, remember to assess the application site both before and after application and to document the procedure appropriately.

Question 134

A nurse is teaching a patient with chronic obstructive pulmonary disease (COPD) how to use a metered-dose inhaler (MDI). Which of the following instructions should the nurse include?

1. Inhale rapidly and deeply when activating the device.
2. Exhale immediately after inhaling the medication.
3. Wait at least 1 minute between puffs if more than one puff is prescribed.
4. Hold the inhaler at least 5 inches away from the mouth.

Answer Key
The correct answer is 3.

Topic: Administration of Inhalation Medications

Inhalation medications are utilized for their local effect on the respiratory system. They are commonly administered through devices such as metered-dose inhalers (MDIs), dry powder inhalers (DPIs), and nebulizers.

Option 3 is correct. If a patient is prescribed more than one puff of the same medication or a different medication, they should wait at least 1 minute between puffs. This allows the first dose to be distributed and absorbed before the second dose is taken.

Option 1 is incorrect. When using an MDI, the patient should breathe in slowly and deeply as they press down on the inhaler, not rapidly. This allows the medication to be carried deeply into the lungs.

Option 2 is also incorrect. After inhaling the medication, the patient should hold their breath for about 10 seconds (or as long as comfortable) to allow the medication to settle in the lungs before exhaling.

Option 4 is incorrect. The MDI should be placed in the mouth, and the mouth should close around it. If using a spacer, the MDI is inserted into one end, and the patient breathes in from the other end.

For the NCLEX, understanding how to correctly administer inhalation medications is critical. Ensure to instruct patients on the importance of correct technique, and remember to assess and monitor the patient's response to the medication. Always follow the five rights of medication administration: right patient, right medication, right dose, right route, and right time.

Question 135

A nurse is preparing to apply a transdermal patch to a patient. Which of the following should the nurse consider when administering transdermal medications?

1. Apply the patch to the same location each time for best absorption.
2. Apply the patch to an area of skin that is hairy, hot, or inflamed.
3. Clean the skin with soap and water before applying the patch.
4. Write the date, time, and nurse's initials on the patch after application.

Answer Key
The correct answer is 3.

Topic: Administration of Transdermal Medications

Transdermal medications are administered via a patch or disk that is applied to the skin. The medication is absorbed through the skin and enters the systemic circulation.

Option 3 is correct. Before applying a transdermal patch, the skin should be clean and dry to ensure optimal absorption of the medication. The use of soap and water to clean the skin is standard practice before applying the patch.

Option 1 is incorrect. You should not apply the patch to the same location each time. Instead, rotate application sites to reduce the risk of skin irritation and enhance absorption.

Option 2 is incorrect. The patch should not be applied to an area of skin that is hairy, hot, or inflamed. These conditions can impede the absorption of the medication. The best locations for patch application are areas with little hair and no damage or inflammation.

Option 4 is not necessarily correct. While some facilities may have this as a policy, it is not a universal standard of care. It's more important to document the location, date, and time of application in the patient's medical record.

On the NCLEX exam, understanding the correct method for applying transdermal patches is vital. They offer several benefits, such as steady release of medication over an extended period, ease of use, and non-invasiveness. However, their effectiveness is highly dependent on proper administration techniques.

Question 136

A nurse is providing education to a client about over-the-counter (OTC) drugs. Which of the following information should the nurse include?

1. OTC drugs can be safely combined with prescription medications without consulting a healthcare provider.
2. OTC drugs do not have side effects.
3. OTC drugs should not be used beyond their expiration date.
4. Using OTC drugs for a prolonged period is safe without healthcare provider supervision.

Answer Key

The correct answer is 3.

Topic: Over the Counter Drug Education and Safety

Over-the-counter (OTC) medications are drugs that can be purchased without a prescription. They are used to treat a variety of minor health issues, from pain and allergies to cold and flu symptoms.

Option 3 is correct. The nurse should inform the client not to use OTC drugs beyond their expiration date. After the expiration date, the drug may not work as expected and could potentially be harmful.

Option 1 is incorrect. Even though OTC drugs are available without a prescription, they can interact with other medications, including prescription drugs. Always consult a healthcare provider before combining OTC and prescription medications.

Option 2 is incorrect. All drugs, including OTC ones, can potentially cause side effects. While these side effects are usually minor, it's important for clients to be aware of them.

Option 4 is incorrect. While some OTC drugs can be used for an extended period, many should not be used long-term without the supervision of a healthcare provider. Prolonged use can lead to issues such as masking the symptoms of a serious condition, developing tolerance, or experiencing side effects.

As an NCLEX candidate, it's crucial to understand the importance of client education related to OTC drugs. Despite their widespread availability and ease of access, these medications should be used responsibly and with awareness of potential risks and interactions.

Question 137

A nurse is monitoring therapeutic drug levels for a client who is on lithium therapy for bipolar disorder. Which of the following symptoms suggests that the client's lithium level may be too high?

1. Hypoactive reflexes.
2. Tinnitus.
3. Fine hand tremors.
4. Diarrhea.

Answer Key
The correct answer is 3.

Topic: Monitoring Therapeutic Drug Levels

Monitoring therapeutic drug levels is a critical part of managing medication therapies for a range of conditions, including mental health disorders like bipolar disorder. Therapeutic drug monitoring involves measuring specific drug concentrations in blood at designated intervals to maintain a constant blood drug concentration.

Option 3 is correct. Fine hand tremors can be a sign of lithium toxicity, suggesting that the lithium levels might be too high. Option 1 is incorrect. Hypoactive reflexes are not typically associated with high lithium levels.

Option 2 is incorrect. Tinnitus, or ringing in the ears, is not a common side effect of lithium.

Option 4 is incorrect. While diarrhea can occur with lithium toxicity, it is less specific and can be caused by many different factors, not only high lithium levels.

As an NCLEX candidate, understanding the importance of monitoring therapeutic drug levels is crucial. Lithium, in particular, has a narrow therapeutic index, meaning the difference between a therapeutic and toxic dose is small.

Regular blood tests are required to ensure the drug stays within the therapeutic range. Signs of toxicity, such as hand tremors, should be promptly reported to the healthcare provider to adjust the dosage as needed.

Question 138

A nurse is implementing a nutritional therapy plan for a client with Crohn's disease. Which of the following recommendations would be the most appropriate for this client?

1. Consume a high fiber diet.
2. Limit fluid intake.
3. Incorporate high-protein foods into the diet.
4. Avoid intake of fruits and vegetables.

Answer Key
The correct answer is 3.

Topic: Nutritional Therapy Implementation

Nutritional therapy involves using specific dietary strategies to promote health, prevent illness, and manage chronic conditions. For clients with Crohn's disease, nutritional therapy plays a crucial role in managing symptoms and reducing inflammation.

Option 3 is correct. Incorporating high-protein foods into the diet is beneficial for clients with Crohn's disease. Protein helps repair body tissues, maintain a healthy immune system, and can aid in recovery during flare-ups.

Option 1 is incorrect. While a high-fiber diet can be beneficial for many individuals, it may not be suitable for clients with Crohn's disease, especially during flare-ups, as it can exacerbate symptoms such as diarrhea and abdominal pain.

Option 2 is incorrect. It's not typically recommended to limit fluids for people with Crohn's disease. Staying hydrated is particularly important for individuals with this condition, as they may be at an increased risk of dehydration due to frequent diarrhea.

Option 4 is incorrect. While some individuals with Crohn's disease may need to avoid certain fruits and vegetables during flare-ups due to their high fiber content, this is not a blanket recommendation for all individuals with the disease. As an NCLEX candidate, it's essential to understand that nutritional therapy must be individualized for each client, considering their specific condition, symptoms, and nutritional needs. For clients with Crohn's disease, the focus should generally be on maintaining a balanced, nutrient-rich diet that avoids personal trigger foods and supports overall health and well-being.

Question 139

A nurse is educating a client who has just started taking the antidepressant MAOI (Monoamine Oxidase Inhibitor). Which of the following foods should the nurse instruct the client to avoid?

1. Baked chicken
2. Fresh fruits
3. Aged cheeses
4. Boiled potatoes

Answer Key
The correct answer is 3.

Topic: Food and Drug Interactions

Understanding food and drug interactions is critical in nursing practice as they can either decrease the effectiveness of medications or potentially cause serious adverse effects.

Option 3 is correct. Clients taking Monoamine Oxidase Inhibitors (MAOIs), a type of antidepressant, should avoid foods high in tyramine. This is because MAOIs inhibit the breakdown of tyramine, a substance found in certain foods, which can lead to dangerously high blood pressure if accumulated. Aged cheeses are known to have high tyramine content and should be avoided.

Option 1, 2, and 4 are incorrect. Baked chicken, fresh fruits, and boiled potatoes are not known to have high levels of tyramine and are generally safe to consume for clients taking MAOIs.

As an NCLEX candidate, you need to recognize the importance of education around food-drug interactions, especially for clients on medications with known dietary restrictions like MAOIs. It's also crucial to teach clients to discuss any dietary concerns with their healthcare provider or a dietitian.

Question 140

A nurse is about to start Total Parenteral Nutrition (TPN) for a client with severe Crohn's disease. Which of the following interventions should be the nurse's priority before initiating the TPN?

1. Checking the client's capillary blood glucose level
2. Verifying the client's last meal
3. Evaluating the client's level of consciousness
4. Confirming placement of the central venous catheter with a chest x-ray

Answer Key
The correct answer is 4.

Topic: Parenteral Nutrition Administration

The administration of Parenteral Nutrition, especially Total Parenteral Nutrition (TPN), is a critical component of managing patients who are unable to maintain adequate nutrition through the gastrointestinal tract, such as severe Crohn's disease.

Option 4 is correct. TPN is typically administered through a central venous catheter due to its high osmolality. Before initiating TPN, the placement of the catheter must be confirmed, usually by a chest x-ray, to avoid complications like pneumothorax, air embolism, or infection. This step is of paramount importance and thus, is the nurse's priority.

Option 1, 2, and 3 are incorrect. While monitoring blood glucose levels is important when administering TPN due to the high glucose content, and evaluating the client's level of consciousness is always crucial, these are not the priority before initiating TPN. Verifying the client's last meal is irrelevant in this case, as TPN is used when oral or enteral feeding is insufficient or not possible.

As an NCLEX candidate, it's important to understand the principles of parenteral nutrition, its indications, and the potential complications. Prioritization and accurate understanding of the interventions related to TPN are key to ensuring patient safety.

Question 141

A nurse is caring for a client who is about to start receiving enteral feedings via a nasogastric tube. Which of the following actions should the nurse perform first?

1. Checking the client's electrolyte levels.
2. Confirming the placement of the nasogastric tube.
3. Warming the formula to room temperature.
4. Providing oral care to the client.

Answer Key
The correct answer is 2.

Topic: Enteral Feeding Administration

Enteral feeding is a strategy used to provide nutrition directly into the gastrointestinal tract through a tube, catheter, or a surgically-created hole into the gut. This is often used when patients cannot consume enough nutrients orally.

Option 2 is correct. Before starting enteral feeding, the most crucial step is to confirm the correct placement of the tube. This is usually done using a combination of methods such as checking pH of aspirate, observing the characteristics of the aspirate, and auscultating while injecting air into the tube. In some settings, radiographic confirmation may be required. Incorrect placement of the tube, especially in the lungs, could lead to serious complications such as aspiration pneumonia.

Option 1, 3, and 4 are not the first actions to be taken. Checking electrolyte levels (option 1) is important when managing patients on enteral feedings as electrolyte imbalances can occur. Warming the formula to room temperature (option 3) can make the feeding more comfortable for the patient, and providing oral care (option 4) is an important part of care for patients on enteral feedings, especially for maintaining oral health and preventing infection.

As an NCLEX candidate, knowing the appropriate steps and sequence of administering enteral feedings can help ensure patient safety and effective delivery of nutrition.

Question 142

A nurse is providing nutritional counseling for a client recently diagnosed with type 2 diabetes. Which of the following information should the nurse include in the teaching plan?

1. Avoid all forms of carbohydrates in the diet.
2. Regular physical activity can help control blood glucose levels.
3. It is not necessary to monitor blood glucose levels at home.
4. Weight gain is expected due to insulin resistance.

Answer Key
The correct answer is 2.

Topic: Nutritional Assessment and Client Education

Nutritional assessment and education is a key component of nursing care, particularly for patients with chronic diseases like type 2 diabetes. As an NCLEX candidate, it's essential to understand the principles of dietary management in diabetes.

Option 2 is correct because regular physical activity is a crucial part of the care plan for a client with type 2 diabetes. Exercise can improve insulin sensitivity and help maintain a healthy weight, both of which can contribute to better control of blood glucose levels.

Option 1 is incorrect. While it's essential to monitor and regulate carbohydrate intake, it's not advisable to avoid all forms of carbohydrates. Carbohydrates are a primary source of energy, and a certain amount is necessary in the diet. The focus should be on consuming complex carbohydrates and avoiding simple sugars.

Option 3 is incorrect. Self-monitoring of blood glucose levels is recommended for clients with diabetes to help manage the disease effectively.

Option 4 is incorrect. Weight gain isn't expected or desired in type 2 diabetes. In fact, weight management is an essential part of managing this disease because obesity is a significant risk factor for insulin resistance.

Teaching should also include information on portion control, meal planning, and the need for regular follow-up with healthcare providers to adjust the care plan as needed.

Question 143

A nurse is educating a client about the use of herbal remedies. The client asks about using St. John's wort for mild depression. Which of the following responses should the nurse provide?

1. "St. John's wort can be effective for mild depression, but you should inform your healthcare provider about its use."
2. "St. John's wort has no known side effects, so it's safe to use."
3. "There's no scientific evidence to support the use of St. John's wort for depression."
4. "As a nurse, I can't provide any information or advice about herbal remedies."

Answer Key
The correct answer is 1.

Topic: Dietary Supplements and Herbal Remedies

As a future NCLEX candidate, it's important to know about dietary supplements and herbal remedies, their uses, potential benefits, side effects, and how they can interact with prescription medications. This information is critical in advising clients and ensuring safe care.

Option 1 is correct. St. John's wort has been studied for its potential benefits in treating mild depression. However, it can interact with several types of medications, including antidepressants, birth control pills, and anticoagulants. Therefore, it's crucial that clients inform their healthcare provider about its use.

Option 2 is incorrect. St. John's wort has several potential side effects, such as dry mouth, dizziness, and gastrointestinal symptoms, and it can also cause photosensitivity. It's not accurate to state that it has no known side effects.

Option 3 is incorrect. There is scientific evidence to suggest that St. John's wort may be beneficial for mild to moderate depression. However, its effectiveness can vary, and it's not recommended for severe depression.

Option 4 is incorrect. As a nurse, it's part of your role to provide education and information about all aspects of health care, including the use of dietary supplements and herbal remedies. However, clients should also be advised to consult with their healthcare provider for personalized advice.

When teaching about herbal remedies, emphasize the need for caution, as these products aren't regulated by the FDA in the same way as prescription medications. The quality, purity, and strength of herbal products can vary significantly, which can affect their safety and effectiveness.

Question 144

A nurse is assisting an elderly client with activities of daily living (ADLs). The client has arthritis and finds it difficult to dress independently. Which of the following interventions should the nurse consider to promote the client's independence?

1. Encourage the client to use adaptive clothing and devices.
2. Insist the client to do all the dressing tasks without help.
3. Advise the client to wait for assistance with all dressing tasks.
4. Recommend the client to avoid dressing altogether to reduce pain.

Answer Key
The correct answer is 1.

Topic: Assisting with Activities of Daily Living

As an NCLEX candidate, understanding how to assist clients with activities of daily living (ADLs), such as dressing, bathing, eating, and mobility, is important. ADLs are essential for a person's well-being and independence.

Option 1 is correct. Adaptive clothing and devices can help clients with physical limitations, like arthritis, to dress more independently. These include clothes with larger buttons or Velcro fasteners, long-handled shoehorns, and dressing sticks.

Option 2 is incorrect. While promoting independence is a goal, insisting a client to do all the dressing tasks without help may lead to frustration, injury, or unnecessary pain, especially if they have conditions like arthritis.

Option 3 is incorrect. While assistance may be necessary for some tasks, promoting independence whenever possible is an important part of care. This might mean providing partial assistance or teaching the client how to use adaptive devices. Option 4 is incorrect. Avoiding dressing altogether is not practical or beneficial for the client. It may lead to decreased independence and self-esteem, and does not promote the client's well-being.

It's important to provide care that encourages self-care abilities and enhances the client's quality of life, while also ensuring their safety and comfort. Tailoring interventions to each client's unique needs and abilities is key to effective nursing care.

Question 145

A nurse is caring for a client who is recovering from hip replacement surgery. Which of the following nursing interventions is most appropriate for promoting physical mobility in this client?

1. Encourage complete bed rest until the surgical wound is healed.
2. Implement passive range of motion exercises in the affected leg.
3. Assist the client in performing active range of motion exercises.
4. Recommend the use of a wheelchair for all mobility.

Answer Key

The correct answer is 3.

Topic: Physical Mobility Promotion

Promoting physical mobility is a crucial aspect of nursing care, particularly in clients who have had surgical procedures that affect their ability to move, such as hip replacement surgery. Option 3 is correct because encouraging the client to perform active range of motion exercises helps to strengthen the muscles, enhance circulation, and improve joint mobility. It is crucial to assist the client as necessary to ensure proper technique and safety.

Option 1 is not the best choice because complete bed rest may lead to muscle atrophy and increase the risk of complications such as deep vein thrombosis and pulmonary embolism. Some movement is usually recommended as soon as possible after surgery, as guided by the healthcare provider.

Option 2 may not be the best choice, as passive range of motion exercises are typically used when clients cannot move on their own. If the client is capable, active participation is usually preferred.

Option 4 is incorrect because overreliance on a wheelchair may discourage the client from using their leg and hinder recovery. While a wheelchair may be necessary in the initial stages or for long distances, the goal should be to improve the client's mobility and independence as much as possible.

Remember, the goal of promoting physical mobility is to help clients regain their strength and independence while ensuring safety. It's essential to collaborate with physical therapists and the client to create a personalized mobility plan that fits the client's needs and abilities. This might include exercises, the use of mobility aids, and regular rest periods.

Question 146

A nurse is caring for a client who had a stroke and now requires a cane for ambulation. Which of the following instructions should the nurse give to the client regarding the use of the cane?

1. Hold the cane on the stronger side of your body.
2. When stepping, move the cane and your weaker leg together.
3. When climbing stairs, lead with the cane, followed by your weaker leg and then your stronger leg.
4. Place your entire weight on the cane when standing from a seated position.

Answer Key

The correct answer is 1, 2, and 3.

Topic: Use of Assistive Devices

Assistive devices such as canes, walkers, and wheelchairs are often used to help individuals who have mobility issues due to various health conditions or injuries. These devices provide support, improve balance, and can promote independence in ambulation.

Option 1 is correct because the cane should be held on the stronger side of the body to provide support to the weaker side.

Option 2 is correct. When walking, the client should first move the cane, then move the weaker leg forward to the level of the cane, and finally, step forward with the stronger leg.

Option 3 is also correct. When climbing stairs, the correct sequence is "up with the good, down with the bad". This means that when going up, the stronger leg should lead, and when going down, the weaker leg should lead.

Option 4 is incorrect. The client should not place their entire weight on the cane when standing from a seated position as it can make the cane unstable and put the client at risk for falls. The proper method involves pushing up from the chair using the arms while keeping the cane on the side of the stronger leg.

As a nurse, it's essential to educate clients on the correct use of assistive devices, and monitor their ability to use the devices safely and effectively. Adjustments to the device, like the height of the cane, might also be necessary for optimal use.

Question 147

A community health nurse is making a home visit to an elderly client who lives alone. Which of the following home safety instructions should the nurse include during the visit?

1. Keep emergency phone numbers in a visible place.
2. Use throw rugs to cover any exposed wiring or cords.
3. Install handrails in the bathroom and on staircases.
4. Store cleaning products in easily accessible locations.

Answer Key

The correct answer is 1 and 3.

Topic: Home Safety Education

Promoting home safety is a crucial part of client education, especially for those at risk for accidents, such as older adults and people with disabilities.

Option 1 is correct. Keeping emergency phone numbers in a visible place is a good practice for all individuals, but especially for those who live alone. These numbers might include local police and fire departments, poison control, and a family member or neighbor.

Option 2 is incorrect. While it's important to manage potential tripping hazards like exposed wires or cords, using throw rugs is not a safe solution. Throw rugs themselves can be a tripping hazard. Instead, wires and cords should be secured and organized in a way that prevents tripping.

Option 3 is correct. Installing handrails in the bathroom (around the toilet and bathtub or shower) and on staircases can provide additional support and prevent falls.

Option 4 is incorrect. Cleaning products, especially those that are toxic or hazardous, should be stored in safe locations out of the reach of children. For older adults, these products should be stored in a manner that doesn't require bending over or reaching up, to prevent falls.

Additional safety measures might include ensuring adequate lighting, keeping walkways clear of clutter, and having functioning smoke and carbon monoxide detectors. Regular home safety assessments can help identify potential hazards and interventions to improve safety.

Question 148

A nurse is providing education to a client who has recently been diagnosed with type 2 diabetes. Which of the following statements by the client indicates understanding of the role of exercise in managing this condition?

1. "I should try to exercise after every meal."
2. "If I start exercising regularly, I can stop taking my medication."
3. "Exercise will help lower my blood sugar levels."
4. "I don't need to monitor my blood sugar levels before and after exercising."

Answer Key

The correct answer is 3.

Topic: Exercise and Activity Education

Educating clients on the importance of exercise and physical activity is a crucial aspect of health promotion and disease prevention. Exercise can help manage various health conditions, including type 2 diabetes.

Option 1 is partially correct. Regular exercise is recommended for individuals with type 2 diabetes, but the timing should be individualized based on the client's medication regimen and blood glucose levels.

Option 2 is incorrect. While regular exercise can contribute to better control of blood glucose levels, it is not a substitute for medication. The client should continue taking their prescribed medications unless advised otherwise by their healthcare provider.

Option 3 is correct. Exercise helps lower blood sugar levels by increasing the body's sensitivity to insulin and promoting more efficient glucose uptake by cells.

Option 4 is incorrect. It is important for individuals with diabetes to monitor their blood sugar levels before and after exercising. Exercise can cause blood sugar levels to drop, which may lead to hypoglycemia. Monitoring blood glucose levels helps to prevent hypoglycemia and ensure that the client's blood sugar levels are within their target range.

It's important to note that before beginning an exercise regimen, the client should have a medical evaluation to determine the type and amount of exercise that is safe and beneficial for them.

Question 149

A nurse is caring for a client who recently underwent a hip replacement surgery. The nurse is preparing to educate the client on the importance of rehabilitation and restorative care. Which of the following information is important for the nurse to include in the teaching?

1. "You can skip physical therapy sessions if you're feeling tired."
2. "It is essential to follow your exercise regimen even when at home."
3. "Pain is an expected part of recovery, and there's no need to report it."
4. "You can start driving as soon as you feel comfortable."

Answer Key
The correct answer is 2.

Topic: Rehabilitation and Restorative Care

Rehabilitation and restorative care are vital in helping individuals regain lost abilities and return to their normal lives after experiencing an illness, surgery, or injury.

Option 1 is incorrect. It's important to adhere to the physical therapy schedule to promote recovery and mobility. If the client feels tired, they should communicate this with their healthcare provider to adjust the rehabilitation program accordingly.

Option 2 is correct. Adherence to the prescribed exercise regimen is crucial for a successful recovery. These exercises help improve mobility, muscle strength, and overall functionality.

Option 3 is incorrect. While some pain is expected during recovery, it should be reported to the healthcare provider. Uncontrolled pain can impede recovery and signal potential complications.

Option 4 is incorrect. Before resuming activities like driving, the client must get clearance from their healthcare provider. Prematurely returning to such activities can put the client at risk for injury.

Question 150

A nurse is preparing a client for surgery. The nurse realizes that the client seems anxious. Which of the following is the most appropriate nursing intervention?

1. Allow the client to make a phone call to a family member for comfort.
2. Administer the prescribed pre-operative medication to reduce the client's anxiety.
3. Tell the client not to worry as it's just a minor procedure.
4. Talk to the client, provide reassurance, and answer any questions about the upcoming surgery.

Answer Key

The correct answer is 4.

Topic: Pre-Operative and Post-Operative Care

Pre-operative and post-operative care are crucial phases in the surgical experience. Nurses play a vital role in both these phases, ensuring clients are physically and psychologically prepared for the surgery and recovery.

Option 1 could be an acceptable intervention if the client specifically requests it, but it doesn't address the root of the anxiety - the client's concerns or lack of understanding about the surgery.

Option 2 is not advisable as it dismisses the client's feelings. Medication is not the only solution for anxiety. Open communication is a better approach.

Option 3 belittles the client's feelings. Regardless of the nature of the procedure, the client's feelings should be validated and addressed professionally.

Option 4 is the most appropriate intervention. It encompasses open communication, education, and emotional support. By discussing the procedure and answering questions, the nurse can help reduce anxiety, make the client feel comfortable, and prepare them for what to expect. Post-operative care focuses on the client's recovery, managing pain, preventing complications, and promoting self-care.

Looking for more practice?

Don't forget to check out
**NCLEX-RN Practice Exam
Part 2: Case Studies**

Available on Amazon

Good luck!

www.ingramcontent.com/pod-product-compliance
Lightning Source LLC
Chambersburg PA
CBHW071443220526
45472CB00003B/648